THE YOGA OF LIFE

THE YOGA OF LIFE

ISAMU MOCHIZUKI

TRANSLATED BY SIMON GRISDALE

authorHOUSE®

AuthorHouse™
1663 Liberty Drive
Bloomington, IN 47403
www.authorhouse.com
Phone: 1-800-839-8640

Published by AuthorHouse   09/19/2012

ISBN: 978-1-4685-8197-3 (sc)
ISBN: 978-1-4685-8198-0 (e)

This book is printed on acid-free paper.

Contents

Lesson Four: Kikō

Foreword

If I am asked if I really believe that Prana exists, I would say that there is no obligation for me to believe in it. I simply feel it.

Prana, an Indian word, is the life-force which fills the universe. It is the energy which keeps us alive, and is emitted in the practice of Yoga. In fact, at first, my own practice of Yoga stemmed from an initial awareness of Prana energy.

When I stood on one leg in a Yoga pose and raised my hands in prayer position above my head, I felt a warm sensation rise up from the Yūsen tsubo (pressure point) in the soles of my feet to the palms of my hands. When I took my hands slightly apart from each other, it felt as if they were alive with electricity.

Again, in poses where I would twist my spine, I detected a fragrant aroma of baked bread.

From these kinds of experiences, I quickly came to the firm realisation that Yoga was much more than merely a set of stretching exercises.

Around that time, I had already been practising Ki therapy, and as I became more and more attracted to Yoga, I felt the need to go to India in order to experience Yoga at its place of origin.

In India, I first stayed at a Hindu temple at the base of the Himalayas, where I practised Yoga poses, breathing exercises and meditation. After that I visited many Yoga practices around the country on foot, and found that each practice and school of teaching differed from each other.

As I began to get a clear idea of the essence of Yoga, I took in as many teachings as I could from these various practices which I found particularly inspiring.

I also became interested in the Japanese Martial Arts and the Chinese methods for developing Ki. Through the practice of Yoga and Ki training, I realised that Yoga has many things in common with Chinese Ki.

From these influences, a style of Yoga linked with Prana gradually took shape. I named this style of Yoga, with its natural assimilation of Ki therapy, 'Prana Yoga'.

By observing the recent global popularity of Yoga, I can see that most of the types belong to the Western style of Yoga. It is practised as an exercise, and even if the poses are from India, the philosophy can only be thought of as Western.

In my opinion, a type of Yoga which is possible for anyone to do, and which enables those who practise it to feel Prana life energy (Ki) is needed.

My aim with this book therefore is to put together a set of Yoga exercises which can be practised not just by healthy people, but also by those who may be elderly, ill, lacking in energy, have stiff joints or dislike sports.

For those who think they are just not designed for Yoga, I would be very glad if you are able to use this book as an opportunity to have a go. You may be surprised how easy it is to feel the life energy which runs through and surrounds us all.

Isamu Mochizuki

Lesson One

Warming Up

Preparation exercises before starting Prana Yoga

Characteristics of Prana Yoga

Prana Yoga is a type of Yoga which integrates Ki into its practice. Anyone of all ages can practise it, and experience Ki (Prana) for themselves. This Yoga is especially effective for those who are stiff.

Furthermore, simple psychological and physical methods of internal control can transform a pose from working on a physical level to a deeper Ki level.

Practising a sequence of Yoga poses is called Asanas (physical method). By practising these Asanas, and enabling the body to bend, curve, stretch and twist, the flow of Ki, or 'Prana' (life energy), will start to flow along the 'Nadi' (also known as the Prana channel, and equivalent to the the Chinese meridians).

Having said that, if these poses are practised merely as a stretching exercise, while muscles may be exercised, the flow of Ki will not be activated. This is the reason why people with illnesses do not see their symptoms improving in spite of practising Yoga.

Here are four things that I have discovered from my experience in helping find suitable Yoga poses for people with illnesses.

1-Perform each movement slowly

When you you pick up speed, the movement becomes an exercise. An important thing to learn is to move your body slowly without using force.

2-Match your movements with your breathing

For example, when you bend forwards, breathe out slowly as you start the movement, and finish your breath at the end of the movement. In the same way, when you breathe in, match your breath with your movement.

Normally we make our movements without thinking about them, so at the start it may be hard to match your movements with your breathing. Persevere though, as it will get easier the more you do it.

3-Concentrate your mind on pain

When you are in a pose and you feel pain, concentrate on the source of pain, and it will occupy your brain cells, and rid your mind of unwanted thoughts. The nerve endings will, during that time, be liberated from any stressful thoughts about work and other matters and make you feel calm and relaxed.

4-When you return to your original position after a pose, take time to savour the effects

When you finish a pose, it is important to return to your original position slowly, taking time to feel your muscles and tendons loosen from their stretched positions. You will become as a result more receptive to the workings of your body, and your concentration will increase.

By doing this, you will also be able to feel the workings of the muscles and organs deep inside the body. Ki will accumulate in the area you direct your attention to, and the circulation of blood around this area will subsequently increase. These deep-level changes in your body will have a positive effect on your health.

Even if the pose is not perfect, if you remember to follow these points, the results will be clear to see. However, if you ignore these points, you cannot expect to receive the age-old benefits of Yoga, no matter how beautiful the pose may look. The difference between Yoga and Stretching is whether or not these points are adhered to or not.

I once had a woman come to me complaining that her illness had not improved even though she had been practising Yoga. After listening to her I understood the reason why. She had thought it was a waste to practise Yoga on its own, so she would watch the television at the same time. By doing this she was not heeding the four points which is clearly why no effect was felt.

The most important pose to do is the relaxing pose

After making a pose in Yoga, it is essential to then relax by doing the relaxing pose, the 'Shava-asana'. Think of this pose as the one designed to make you relax. If you feel comfortable and relaxed, then you have practised Yoga properly.

By the same rationale, even if you can do many poses including the difficult ones perfectly, if you don't do a pose for relaxing afterwards, (or do not feel relaxed even after doing it) then you cannot say you have practised Yoga properly.

You may find this surprising, but in fact the most difficult pose out the hundreds of poses there are in Yoga is the relaxing pose.

So what does it actually mean to relax? The 're' from 'relax' means 'again' and the 'lax' comes from Latin and means 'loosen'. The literal meaning of 'relax' is therefore to 'loosen again'. What then do we have to 'loosen again'?

It is said that we feel tension from the time we learn how to speak, view the world and start to conceive time. From this we can deduce that we can only start to experience true relaxation in a state of consciousness where there is no perception of time.

A state of consciousness where there is no perception of time corresponds to a baby before it learns how to speak, to animism. 'Re' from 'relax' means to once 'again' return to a mind without time, in other words to the Universe itself. 'Relax' therefore means to become one with the Universe.

Originally, the relaxing pose is a profoundly deep aspect of Yoga, designed as a means of becoming at one with the Universe.

One more important benefit from relaxing is that it restores the balance of the autonomic nerves. This is crucial because it is believed that in retaining balance between the sympathetic nerves and the para-sympathetic nerves almost all illnesses can be cured.

Recently, there was a landmark discovery in immunology research when the autonomic nerves were seen to control white blood cells. According to an immunology research paper by Professor Tōru Abo of Niigata University, only three percent of illnesses are attributed to our genes and the remainder are all due to the imbalance in the autonomic nerves. If we can therefore relax through Yoga and restore the balance in the autonomic nerves, we should be able to cure almost any illness.

The key to Prana exercises

Let us now start the Yoga lesson and experience this deep relaxation for ourselves. There is no need for any particular preparation for Yoga, but please wear clothes which are not too tight and practise barefoot.

To warm up before starting Yoga first loosen any stiffness in your muscles. Here is a Prana exercise for that purpose which anyone can do.

When practising Prana or Yoga, make sure it is at least one hour after you have eaten. If you practise just after eating, you may feel nauseous. If your body is very warm such as after taking a bath or shower, then wait until you have cooled down.

Another thing to remember is not to get up quickly after relaxing. There are people who get up sprightly, but this is not a good habit to have. The relaxing pose is called Shava-asanas, which means in Sanskrit 'the corpse pose'. The body is so deep in relaxation it is almost as if it is dead, which is why you must move your hands and feet to first signal to the body you are getting up before picking yourself up slowly.

Prana Exercises

Releasing stagnant energy through arm and leg Asanas (poses)

1- Sit down with your legs in front of you, and bend your toes back and forth ten times.

Next, bend your ankles back and forth ten times.

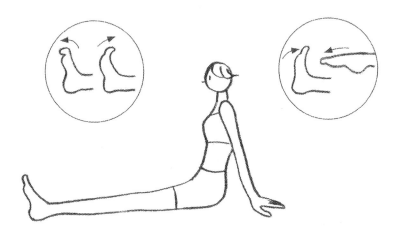

2- Spread your legs a little, and turn your right ankle inwards ten times. Now turn it outwards ten times. Do the same with your left ankle.

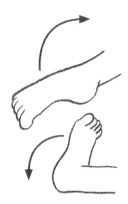

3- Bend your right leg and place it on your left thigh. Place your left hand with each of your fingers in between your toes, and turn the ankle ten times in one direction, then ten times again in the other.

Do the same with your other leg.

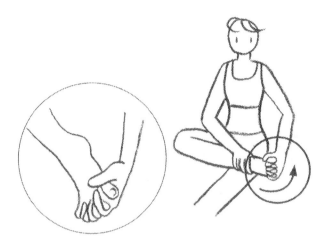

4- With your left hand hold your right ankle and bounce your right knee ten times with your right hand, so you feel the stretch in your hip joint.

Do the same with your left leg.

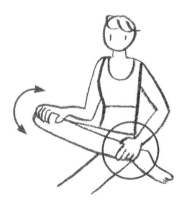

5- Join the soles of your feet together, bouncing both knees ten times so you feel the stretch in your hip joints.

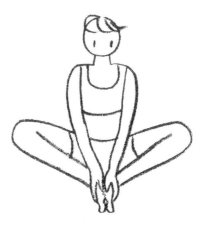

6- Cross your legs and hold your hands behind your back.

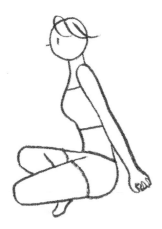

7- Stretch your arms out straight and breathe in. As you do so, bring your arms and chin up then hold your breath in this stretched position.
You should feel the stretch around your shoulder blades.
Return to the original position while breathing out.

Do this twice.

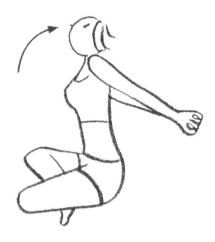

8- Stretch your legs out in front of you and hold your hands behind your head. While breathing in, bring your hands up then hold your breath in this position. Return to the original position while breathing out.

Do this twice.

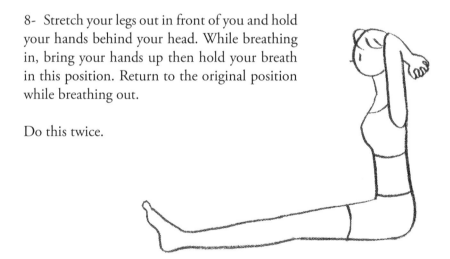

9- Do the movement a third time, but this time after you breathe in and raise your hands up, lean your outstretched arms to the right, stretching your left side while breathing out.

Return your arms to the original position while breathing in, then lean your arms to the left, stretching your right side while breathing out.

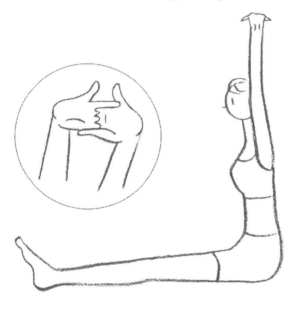

10- Return your arms to the original position while breathing in, then release your hands and bring them down to your side while breathing out.

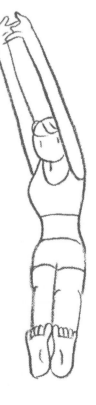

11- Raise your shoulders while breathing in, then exhale and drop them quickly. Repeat this four to five times.

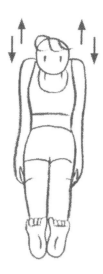

Relax in the Shava-asana pose (See next page)

Notes:

These arm and leg exercises prepare the body and mind for Yoga by activating the channels of Ki in the body (Keiraku) and releasing stagnant energy.

These exercises are suitable for the weak, ill and elderly, and can improve the health of an individual when practised on their own.

Shava-asana

Enables deep relaxation

- Close your eyes, turn your palms upwards, and breathe out slowly. Focus on your out breath- imagine you are breathing out from your fingertips and toes. You don't need to focus on your in breath- just let the air enter your lungs naturally: your stomach will automatically fill up with the same amount of air that leaves.

- Lie flat on your back and keep your legs the same distance apart as your shoulders.

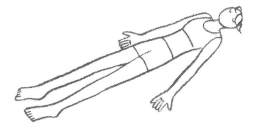

- Move your hands and legs before slowly getting up.

Notes:

Use this pose to relax your whole body after moving. Your breathing will become relaxed, improving your blood circulation and enabling oxygen to be passed all around the body.

When you do this pose, imagine the peaceful sensation of your whole body sinking into the floor.

Column 1

The origin of Yoga

The origin of the term Yoga is the Sanskrit term Yui, meaning to tie a horse to a cart.

There are scholars who believe that the term goes back as far as the Indus civilization which prospered five thousand years ago. In the valley of the River Indus are two large archaeological remains, Mohenjo-daro and Harappa, from which seated figures in poses and in meditation have been discovered.

These discoveries suggest that from ancient times, man has always sought ways to control his mind. Indeed, it is said that the term Yoga was used because of the similarity in nature of using a method to control the incessant ramblings of the mind and a driver tying his horse to his cart.

No doubt Yoga was seen as the most superior technique for controlling the human mind as it became commonplace for the religious practitioners in India where six schools of Yoga evolved.

1- Rāja Yoga (lineage from classical Yoga, with emphasis on mind control)

2- Bhakti Yoga (devotion)

3- Karma Yoga (selfless service)

4- Jnana Yoga (philosophical contemplation)

5- Mantra Yoga (reciting incantations)

6- Hatha Yoga (physiological discipline)

Today, Yoga is not just practiced in India but all over the world. When I studied Yoga at temples in the Himalayas, I was joined by Hindus, Buddhists, Muslims, Judaists, and Christians from the West. Within

Christianity nowadays, there is also 'Christian Yoga', a discipline designed to deepen worship.

The Yoga most of us know about is number six, Hatha Yoga. The founder is said to be Gorakhnath, a holy man who lived in the beginning of the thirteenth century. 'Hatha' means 'power'. It is the most approachable type of Yoga, with the most immediate physical benefits.

Lesson Two

Morning Yoga

Morning poses for feeling lively throughout the day

The key to morning Yoga

It is especially beneficial to practise Yoga in the morning. By doing these exercises, Prana, life-force energy which fills the air around us, can be inducted into the body, making us feel lively throughout the day.

When doing the Sun Worship pose (p.17), face the east and imagine a bright red early morning sun rising up in front of you.

Always remember to match your breathing with your movements. Imagine you are taking in the sun's energy when you breathe in and getting rid of waste matter and stagnant energy when you breathe out.

Your day can be decided by how you conduct the morning. When you have time to spare, practise breathing exercises, meditation and an affirmation exercise after the Sun Worship pose.

The affirmation exercise involves declaring a positive statement. Say aloud three times phrases such as 'today I am feeling great again', 'I feel totally refreshed', or 'everything went well in every way'.

You may not notice any difference at the beginning, but if you continue with it, the great power that can be generated from such a simple declaration will become apparent to you.

Exercise Schedule

When you are feeling lively in the morning, practise these in order:

◆ Sun Worship pose ×2 (p.17)

◆ Shava-asana (p.12)

◆ Re-energizing breathing exercise (p.95)

◆ Mantra Breathing Meditation technique (p.111)

◆ Affirmation exercise (p.15)

When you feel sleepy in the morning, practise these in order:

◆ Opening the chest out from prayer position pose (p.22)

◆ Shava-asana (p.12)

Sun Worship pose

How to bring the Prana energy rich in the air around us into the body

1- Stand up straight with your feet together, and join your palms together in prayer position in front of your chest. Keep your breathing slow and even.

2- When you breathe in, stretch your arms back and hold your breath. Make sure your elbows are straight.

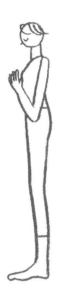

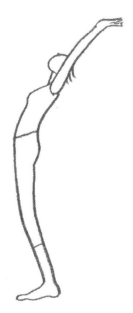

3- While exhaling, bend your top half down and hold your breath when the palms of your hands are on the floor either side of your feet.

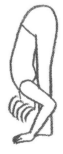

4- While holding your breath with your palms on the floor, stretch your left leg out behind you and raise your foot onto your toes. Breathe in, then keeping your left knee and your fingertips on the floor, raise your head and bend back as far as you can. Hold your breath at the end of the inhalation.

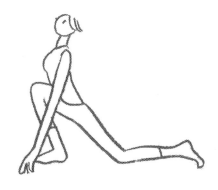

5- While holding your breath, place your palms firmly on the floor, extend your elbows then stretch your right leg, then your left leg behind you, so that your head, body and legs are in a straight line.

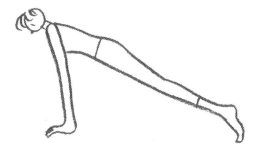

6- While exhaling, bend both elbows and lower your knees, chest and forehead onto the floor until the end of your breath. Raise your bottom up a little as you do so.

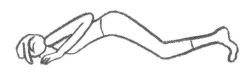

7- While breathing in, lower your stomach onto the floor, extend your elbows and raise your head.
When your arms are straight and you have stretched back as much as you can, hold your breath in this position.

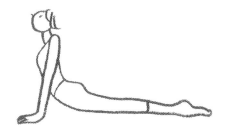

8- While exhaling, straighten both arms and legs, keep the soles of your feet firmly on the floor, stick your bottom in the air and hold your breath at the end of the exhalation.

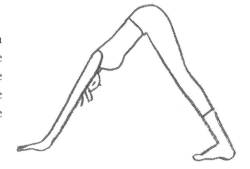

9- While holding your breath, bend your left knee, and move your left leg up inside both arms.
Bend your right knee onto the floor, breathe in and bend back as much as you can, holding your breath in this position at the end of the inhalation. (This is the same as (4) with your legs interchanged)

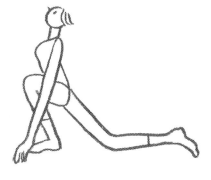

10- While holding your breath, place both palms on the floor and bring your right foot up next to your left foot. While exhaling, straighten both legs, bend the top half of your body down onto your legs, and hold your breath at the end of the exhalation. (The same as (3))

11- Breathe in slowly, take your palms off the floor, raise them up in the air and stretch your arms back. Hold your breath at the end of the inhalation. (The same as (2))

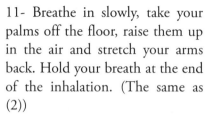

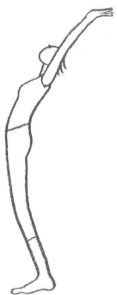

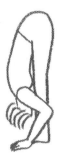

12- While exhaling, return to an upright standing position, briefly joining your hands in prayer position before lowering them to your side. Rest a short while before doing this once more.

Relax in the Shava-asana pose

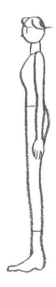

Notes:

When practising the Sun Worship pose, you are expressing your gratitude to the glory of the sun. This dynamic series of poses uses the whole body and only need a short space of time to refresh both the body and mind. They are thus perfect to do at the start of the day. It only takes about three minutes to do all the poses, so please practise them every morning.

If you look behind you when you bend back in poses 2 and 11, you will find you can stretch easier.

In poses 4 and 9 where you stretch your leg behind you, fix your ankle in front firmly on the floor to prevent it rising up, keep your upper body up straight and make sure you stretch your back.

When you bend the top half of your body back in 7, keep your legs together when you stretch, , and try to keep your thighs and feet firmly on the floor.

In 8, if you keep your head between your arms, it will be easier to stretch your back. Also, if you make sure your ankle does not rise above the floor, your knee will stretch more.

Opening the chest out from prayer position

Effective on its own for people who find it hard to get up in the morning

1- Go into the kneeling position and put your palms together in front of your chest in prayer position. Breathe silently.

2- Breathe in, and with your palms together, raise your arms up slowly, holding your breath at the end of the inhalation when your arms feel they have gone high enough.

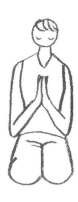

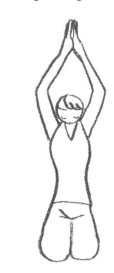

Make a fist with your hands by folding each finger over the thumb.

3- While holding your breath, release your palms, and open your arms out.

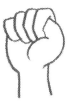

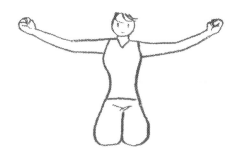

4- Keep holding your breath, and bend your head backwards.

Bring your arms back behind you and open your chest out.

Bend your wrists in and twist them around.

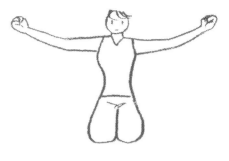

5- While breathing out, bend the top half of your body down and bend your arms back behind you while keeping your hands in fists. Bring your arms up high behind you and hold your breath at the end of the exhalation when your forehead touches the floor.

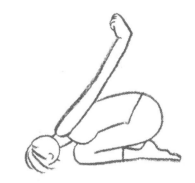

6- When you breathe in, raise your body up. Bring your arms back down in front of you, and place your palms together in prayer position again in front of your body.

After making a breath, repeat the pose two to three times.

Relax in the Shava-asana pose

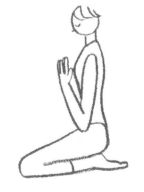

Notes:

In the pose where the chest is expanded from prayer position, moving the top half of the body backwards and forwards pumps the old blood accumulating in the stomach back into the heart, and replaces it with fresh new blood. This improves the blood circulation in the body, making you feel more energized.

Those who find it hard getting out of bed should practise this pose while sitting on the bed. As you do the pose numerous times, you will notice your head becoming clearer, and you will feel more energetic.

When you master this pose, on (6) be aware of your palms as you place them together in front of your chest. As your palms get closer together, you should start to feel a warmth radiating between your hands. The moment the palms touch it will feel like a discharge of static electricity is running between them, When your palms are completely joined together, it will feel as if everything around has disappeared and all that exists now in the universe is the warmness in your hands.

Column 2

The power of Affirmation

Someone I know overcame depression merely by saying the word 'no' with a strong resolve.

Back then she was still a young housewife. One day, she hit her car into a cyclist. Immediately she got out of the car and asked him if he was all right, but the man had already picked himself and his bike up. He had glared at the car for some time before leaving in silence.

At the time she was very relieved, but when she got home, she couldn't get the image of hitting the cyclist out of her mind. And from there the worries started to mount. She wondered if the cyclist was indeed hurt, or if he had remembered her number plate since she she had been looking at it, which would mean she would hear about it soon. She also started to worry that the man would pretend he had been injured, and extort a large amount of money from her. In this way her mind kept on playing out the various worst case scenarios until she began to feel very down.

Times of strife tend to bring up bad memories. The woman suddenly remembered a TV program she watched long ago in which a loan shark deliberately crashes into someone's car and demands the driver hand out money for medical fees. Now she had trouble sleeping at night. No matter what she was doing, if she was awake, or sleeping, she was overrun with her fears. Eventually her mental state became so severe that she wondered if it would be better to end her life.

It was in this state of depression that she came to my clinic for treatment. When the young housewife told me she couldn't sleep at night, I could see in her eyes the fear of being chased down by something.

After I had administered Ki and she had become very relaxed, I advised her to do the following. 'If an unpleasant thought enters your mind, just say 'no' strongly in your mind. Merely asserting 'no' will prevent the unpleasant thought or waveform from entering your mind and make it disappear.'

She tried this out and discovered that indeed, just by saying 'no', her anxieties disappeared.

Now the woman enjoys a peaceful state of mind and lives a happy life.

Lesson Three

Prana Yoga
Reinvigorating Yoga

The secret of Prana Yoga

I will now explain the poses we do at my Yoga class in order. First relax yourself with the Prana exercises. Ki is incorporated in the areas in the body which are relaxed from doing Yoga and this improves the Ki channels in the body. Practising Yoga, Ki and breathing exercises equally will release tension in the body and alleviate tiredness.

To relax is important for this style of Yoga. Between each pose we will always rest in the Shava-asana pose.

After the Ki exercises, please try and gather Ki yourselves with the method used on pages 82-84.

To carry out all the Prana Yoga exercises takes about an hour. For those who don't have this much time to spare please refer to the following chart.

Women should add to this the Cat pose, which improves the function of hormones.

Exercise Schedule:

When you have time, practise these in order:

- ◆ Prana exercises (p.6)

- ◆ Poses from the Diamond pose (1) to the Cat pose (13)

- ◆ Sun Worship pose (p.17)

- ◆ Leg Ki exercise 1,2,3 and 4 (p.73-80)

- ◆ Ki collecting method (p.82)

- ◆ Bending forward with legs astride pose (14)

- ◆ Standing on the head pose (20)

- ◆ Single nostril breathing exercise A, B, Re-energizing breathing exercise , Depression alleviating breathing exercise, Refreshing breathing exercise, Brain breathing exercise for insomnia (p.93-103)

- ◆ Shava-asana (p.12)

When you don't have time, practise these in order:

- ◆ Prana exercises (p.6)

- ◆ Head-to-knee pose (5)

- ◆ The Camel pose (10)

- ◆ Spine-twisting pose (11) and, for women only, the Cat pose (13)

- ◆ Shava-asana (p.12)

(1) The Diamond pose

The basic way to sit in Yoga

1- Kneel down, slide your feet and lower legs together, and lay your feet flat on the floor with toes pointing straight out behind you. Sit back onto your heels. Keep your chin in a little and imagine that the top of your head is being pulled up.

2- Relax your neck, shoulders, upper arms, elbows and wrists. Relax your palms and all the fingers.

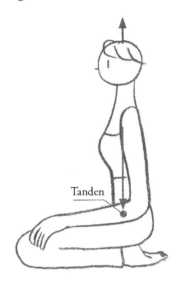

3- When you relax your upper body, your weight will be taken by the stomach. Concentrate on the 'tanden' (the area five centimetres under the navel).

4- Keep the big toes at touching distance- refrain from overlapping the feet. Rest your arms lightly on your lap. Keep your back straight.

5- Close your eyes, and regulate your breathing. Continue this for one to two minutes.

Notes:

In this pose the top half of the body is kept light and relaxed, while the bottom half is kept firm and stable as if rooted to the floor. When you feel your weight bearing on your stomach, be aware of this feeling. It should be relatively low down and will start to heat up when you focus on it. This is your 'tanden'.

(2) Bending forward whilst kneeling pose

Corrects any misalignments in the body

1- From the diamond pose, place your hands on the floor in front.

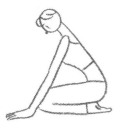

2- While breathing out, bring the stomach in, lower the head and curve the back until the end of the exhalation.

3- When you breathe in, bring your head up and straighten your back while keeping your hands on the floor until the end of the inhalation.

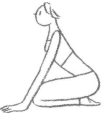

4- While exhaling, stretch your arms out forwards on the floor as far as you can and hold your breath in this position.

You should feel a good stretch in your arms and back.

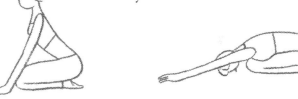

5- Breathe in and bring your hands back in front of you while finishing the inhalation, then return to the diamond pose while breathing out. Repeat 1-5 twice.

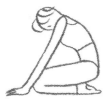

The second time around, when stretching your arms in front of you in (4), stay in this position for a short while and breathe normally.

For those who want to feel more of a stretch in their arms, shoulders, or back, bend your head down diagonally when doing (4) for the second time. Continue with the following pose which stretches the right and left side of the body.

(3) Pose for stretching the right and left sides of the torso

Practise after the Bending forward whilst kneeling pose

1- From the diamond pose, place both hands on the floor next to your left knee. Put your wrists together, with your right hand pointing in front and your left hand pointing backwards.

2- While exhaling, bring your stomach in, lower your head and curve your back until you reach the end of the exhalation.

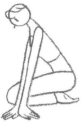

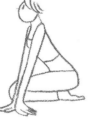

3- While breathing in, lift your head up and bend backwards until you reach the end of the inhalation.

5- Breathe in, and return both hands to their original position as you end your inhalation. Breathe out while returning to the diamond pose.

4- While breathing out, stretch your right arm out in front and your left arm behind, keeping your hands on the floor, and at the end of the exhalation, hold your breath in this position. Keep your right ear on your right arm so that both arms feel they are being stretched.

6- Repeat this with the right side.

Practise this twice each side. The second time around, when your arms are outstretched on the floor, stay in this position for a short while and breathe naturally.

Relax in the Shava-asana pose.

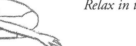

Notes:

Misalignment of the jaw and the teeth can be corrected by stretching the upper body forwards and sideways in this pose. When doing this pose, some find that one arm is flexible and the other stiff. Sometimes this corresponds to the misalignment of the jaw or teeth. If you find this is the case with you, start the pose with the flexible side and end with the stiff side.

If the pose is practised the other way round, the flexible side will become even more flexible, and the misalignment will get worse. Those with poor balance between right and left should do the pose for the stiff side an extra time.

When both sides are as flexible as each other, this should indicate that the misalignment is corrected.

Here is a story of someone who had been practising this pose. One day at meal time, he found he had problems chewing his food when suddenly his false tooth fell out. Originally the alignment of his teeth had been poor, and this had been adjusted with the insertion of a false tooth. According to his dentist, the misalignment had corrected itself, causing the false tooth to collide with the other teeth and come loose.

With this experience the man realised that general misalignments of the body can correspond to misalignments in specific parts of the body.

(4) Lying back and kneeling pose

Regulates the movement of the stomach and bowels

1- From the diamond pose separate your heels so that your bottom is on the floor.

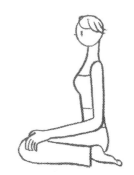

2- Using your elbows, slowly lower your upper body down onto the floor behind you.

3- Join your hands on your stomach and relax your body.

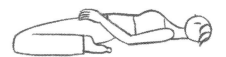

4- Straighten your arms on the floor above your head then extend both arms while breathing in. Breathe naturally at the end of the inhalation. Give your back a comfortable stretch as you do this.

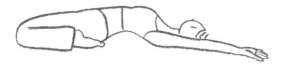

5- Join your hands on the stomach again, rest your eyes and breathe silently for two to three minutes.

Relax in the Shava-asana pose

Notes:

Those with painful knees should wait until they are better before doing this pose.

Those with a stiff back should at the start put a cushion behind their back and lower themselves down gradually into the pose.

Note that this pose can also be practised straight after a meal. This has beneficial effects for those who have problems with their stomach or bowels.

In (3) when you relax with your hands together on your stomach, you should feel a pleasant sensation of something pressed against a part of your lower back. This is where the stomach and bowel 'tsubo' (pressure point) is, and stimulating it in this pose will improve the health of these organs.

If, say, at a party, you overeat and you feel bloated, try this pose. As if like magic, this bloated feeling will disappear. Be careful though; if you eat again as a result, you will put on weight.

(5) Head-to-knee pose

Strengthens the internal organs and lower back

1- Sit on the floor, spread your legs out, then bend your left leg so that your left heel is right against your body.

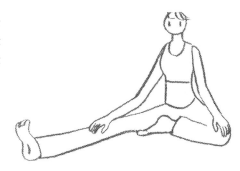

2- Stretch both arms out and hold your big right toe with your index finger and thumb of your right hand, with your left hand on top.

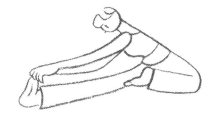

3- Breathe out slowly while bringing in your stomach and curving your back.

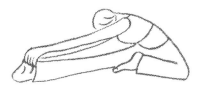

4- While breathing in, bring your lower back in, bring your chin up, and stretch your arms, holding your breath at the end of the inhalation.

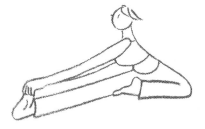

5- Breathe out and while relaxing your chin and lower back, bend forwards and touch your forehead onto your right knee as you come to the end of your exhalation. Hold your breath here.

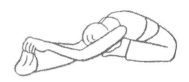

6- As you breathe in, return to the original pose, bringing your upper body up and releasing your hands from the big toe of your right foot as you finish the inhalation.

Take a little breather, then practise the pose again. The second time around, when you finish the exhalation in (5), breathe normally and stay in this position for a moment. Do the same again with the left side.

Relax in the Shava-asana pose

Notes:

The Head-to-knee pose is one of the most important forward bending poses. If you are unable do this pose well, you will also find it hard to do the other poses well.

Those who cannot reach their big toe can start from where they can reach on the ankle. It is important however to make sure that your knee is locked and firmly on the floor.

This pose strengthens the inner organs and lower back by stimulating all the organs in the abdomen.

(6) The Fish pose

Opens out the rib cage, and improves lung function

1- Lie down, face up. Put your legs together and stretch them out. Place your arms alongside your body, palms up.

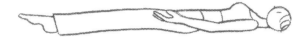

2- As you breathe in, put your weight on your elbows and push up. As your chest rises, let your neck bend back as far as you can. Hold your breath at the end of the inhalation and breathe naturally in this position for ten to twenty seconds. Your chest is at this stage supported by three points; your head, elbows and bottom.

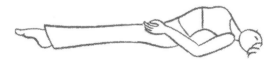

Relax in the Shava-asana pose

Notes:

It is important when practising the Fish pose to relax both legs. When you get used to the pose you will need just the head and bottom to lift your chest up without having to use your elbows. Doing the pose in this way will strengthen the neck, making it more stable for when you do the head stand pose.

The pose opens the chest out, enabling deep breathing and improving the function of the lungs. It is effective against asthma and other breathing ailments.

It also improves posture, and can combat round shoulders.

(7) Gas reduction pose

Stimulates the digestive organs and works against constipation

1- Lie down on the floor with your legs stretched out together, facing upwards.

2- Bend your right leg and bring it up to your body, and join your hands around your shin. Keep your left leg outstretched, and relaxed.

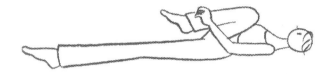

3- While breathing out, use both arms to bring your thigh to your chest. At the same time, bring your torso up from the floor and finish your exhalation as your chin touches your knee. Hold your breath in this position for ten seconds.

4- As you exhale, relax your arms and bring your leg and body back down onto the floor.
Practise both sides twice, one side after the other.

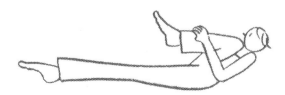

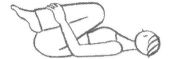

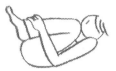

5- While breathing out, bend your legs and bring them up with your hands around your shins, finishing your exhalation as your chin touches your knees. Hold your breath in this position for ten seconds.

As you breathe in, relax both arms and bring both legs and upper body back down onto the floor. Practise this twice.

Relax in the Shava-asana pose

Notes:

In the Gas Reduction pose, make sure you have fully exhaled the air in your lungs as your chin touches your knee/s. By doing so, your stomach will draw in, and your thighs will put pressure on your intestines, stimulating your digestive organs.

This pose is effective for those who suffer from a bloated stomach or constipation.

(8) The Standing Tree pose

Improves balance and concentration

1- Stand up straight with your toes and heels together in line.

2- Bend your right leg, and hold your right ankle up with your right hand, so that the heel is firmly fixed in the inside of your left leg.

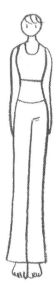

3- Put your hands in prayer position in front of your chest.

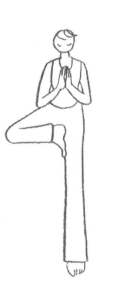

4- Raise your hands as you breathe in until your arms are against your ears, and hold your breath at the end of the inhalation.

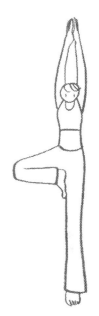

5- Breathe naturally, and stay balanced in this pose. You cannot control your balance like this if you have your eyes closed, so keep your eyes on a point diagonally in front of you on the floor, and you will be able to stay stable. Start by holding this position for ten seconds, then increase to 20 seconds, then 30 seconds and so on.

6- As you breathe out, lower your hands silently back in front of your chest, and breathe naturally.
Release your hands from the prayer position and silently lower your right leg back down to the original position in (1).
Now do the pose for your left leg.

Relax in the Shava-asana pose

Notes:

For the Standing Tree pose, it is important to make sure that when you are standing on one leg and start to wobble, you do not grab hold of something to steady you, such as the wall or a pillar. When you balance on one leg, the muscles in the sole of the foot will move in order to achieve balance. These movements are what makes this pose effective.

Grabbing hold of a pillar may make it easier to hold the pose, but will eliminate any movement in the sole of the foot.

If you wobble but try hard to stay stable, an inner power in the body is activated which through practice can be controlled.

If you practise this every morning, you will discover there are days when you can do it perfectly and days when you find it difficult. This can reveal the state of your biorhythm. On days you find it difficult to balance in the pose, you should take extra care in activities such as driving.

For those who have time, try practising the pose for two minutes in total: one minute for each leg. Research by a certain doctor discovered that two minutes of the pose was equivalent to the energy expended in a thirty minute walk.

By transferring all of the body weight on one leg, the cells in the bones are strengthened, preventing osteoporosis and lessening the probability of breakages in accidents.

Column 3

The Standing Tree pose develops super-human abilities

In India there are some people who practise the Standing Tree pose for half or all of the day in order to develop superhuman abilities. For most of us who do not have the time to do this, twenty seconds or more is sufficient. In the past, the British television company the BBC showed a feature on a Yogi in India who had practised the Standing Tree pose continually for decades. He had his leg tied up and at night he hung on to a swing as he slept, while in the morning his disciple carried him to the river to bathe him. However, the program did not get round to testing any superhuman abilities he may have had.

The soles of the feet are vital in the makeup of the body. This is something I realised from a program I watched once on TV. First, they showed an archery master shoot an arrow at a target. The arrow hit the target as if it was magnetized. Next he put adzuki beans in his socks and shot at the target again. This time the arrow missed the target. Finally he put grains of rice in his socks and shot at the target. He missed the target again, although not as much as with the adzuki beans. The slight stimulus from the adzuki beans and rice grains on the soles of his feet had evidently weakened the powers of intuition. I thus came to the understanding from watching this that the ends of the limbs are in fact connected to the brain.

(9) Back-stretching pose

Eliminates anxiety by stimulating the para-sympathetic nerves

1- Sit down, with your legs outstretched together in front of you.

2- Clasp both big toes with each index finger and thumb.

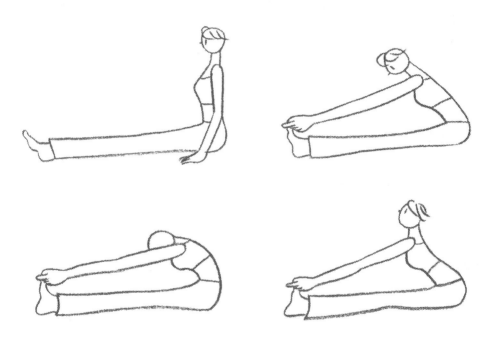

3- While breathing out, draw your stomach in and hunch your back until the end of the exhalation.

4- While breathing in, arch your back and stretch your arms. Extend your chin and chest out so that as you come to the end of your inhalation you are looking at the ceiling.

5- While breathing out, lower your torso down to the floor so that your stomach, chest and face are touching your legs as you come to end of the exhalation.

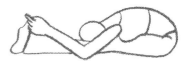

6- While breathing in, lift your torso up, release your hands from your toes and at the end of the inhalation breathe naturally, returning to the original position in (1). Repeat this twice, breathing naturally for a short while in (5) when doing it the second time around.

Relax in the Shava-asana pose

Notes:

It is important to keep your legs straight, so if you find your knees bob up when reaching for your toes, reach for your ankles or an area further up your leg. When you have made the pose, imagine that your body is connected all the way down, from your neck to your back, to your thighs down to your Achilles tendon. This pose puts pressure on the stomach, improving the activity of all the inner organs.

If practised before going to bed, the stimulation of the para-sympathetic nerves will make anxieties disappear, and calm the mind.

(10) The Camel pose

Works against stiff shoulders and stooped upper back

1- Kneel down in the diamond pose (p.28).

2- Put two fists in between your knees to separate them then raise yourself up on your toes.

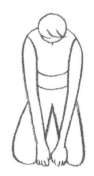

3- Place both hands on your hips, then breathe in slowly while extending your chest out and bending your body and head back.

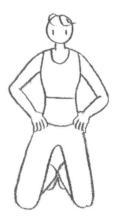

4- Silently release you hands from your hips and let them hang down towards your ankles. Press the palms of your hands firmly against the soles of your feet.

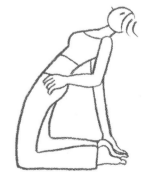

5- Breathe naturally as your palms are pressed onto the soles of your feet, then breathe out as you bend back and extend your chest and thighs. Stick your chin out and bend your neck back as far as you can, breathing naturally in this position.

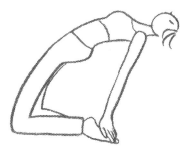

6- Breathe out slowly, releasing your hands from your feet, and returning them to your waist. Raise your body back up, until it is straight and you are in the kneeling position again.

Repeat this pose twice.

Relax in the Shava-asana pose

Notes:

Those who are stiff should not force their bodies in order to achieve the pose. Start with your knees wide apart and gradually practise with them closer together. Once you have become used to the pose, try it with your knees touching each other. Those who become proficient with the pose will find their bodies will slack when breathing out in (5). In this case try extending the waist out further as it will get more flexible as a result.

This pose opens out the chest and helps prevent hunched shoulders. It also improves the blood circulation of the liver, kidneys, adrenal gland and pancreas and is effective against obesity, rheumatism and diabetes.

(11) Spine-twisting pose

Helps the spine become flexible and eliminates fatigue

1- Sit down and stretch your legs out in front of you. Bend your left knee so that your heel is pressed against your body. Hook your right index finger around your right big toe, and place your left palm on the left side of your body.

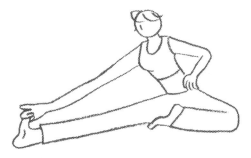

2- Facing the front, breathe in slowly, then twist your body round to the left. First, twist your neck as far as it will go, then follow with the shoulders and lower back until the end of the inhalation.

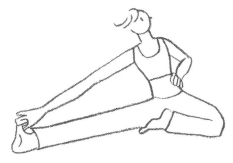

3- Breathe out slowly and return to the original position. Repeat this once more. The second time around, breathe naturally at (2), and stay in this pose for a short while.

4- Do the same for the right leg.

Relax in the Shava-asana pose

Notes:

Try and feel each section of vertebrae when you twist the different parts of the body: for the neck, feel the cervical (top of the spine) vertebrae, for the shoulders, the thoracic (mid-spine) vertebrae, and for the lower back the lumber (lower spine) vertebrae. When you breathe naturally the second time around, concentrate on your spine. Imagine a pleasant sensation in your neck, chest, and lower back while you twist.

This pose will increase flexibility and correct misalignments in the spine and will also have an immediate effect in relieving tiredness. In addition, by doing this simple pose, and increasing flexibility in the spine, a sensory perception of what is behind you can be achieved. This came in very handy for someone I know when he found himself in a threatening situation.

He had been in a taxi waiting at the traffic lights when suddenly he felt an unpleasant feeling in his spine. Immediately he stuck his legs out stiffly, tucked in his chin and lay down with his head firmly pressed on the back seat support. Moments later, a car collided into the back of the taxi. Even though serious whiplash injuries would normally be incurred from such a collision, the man escaped unharmed. He sees his fortunate outcome as proof of the benefits of practising Yoga.

(12) The Triangle pose

Corrects misalignments of the spine and is effective against Scoliosis

1- Stand up with your legs wide apart (at an angle of about 40 degrees). Keep your arms flat against your side.

2- Breathe in, lift up both arms, turn both palms downwards and stretch your arms and shoulders horizontally outwards until the end of the inhalation.

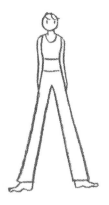
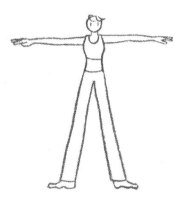

3- Turn your right palm up, then turn your head to the right and look at your palm.

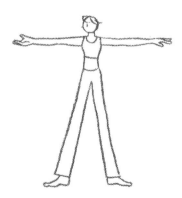

4- Exhale and stretch your straightened arm above your head to the left, keeping your eye on your right palm. Move your left hand down your left leg as your right arm touches your ear and curves to make a circle, becoming parallel to the floor. Come to the end of the exhalation as the upper arm touches your ear and hold your breath in this position for five seconds.

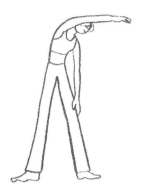

5- As you breathe in, do the pose in reverse so you arrive back at (1).

6- Next, do the same for the left arm. Repeat the pose twice, one side after the other. The second time around breathe naturally at (4), staying in this position for ten seconds.

Relax in the Shava-asana pose

Notes:

When stretching the body to the side, be careful not to draw your back in. You will find the side of your body will stretch easier when your back sticks out a touch.

The Triangle Pose can be practiced as effective treatment against Scoliosis. Those who have one side more flexible than the other should start with the flexible side and end with the stiffer side. If the difference in flexibility between the sides is considerable, practise the pose an extra time for the stiff side. Once both sides become equally flexible this will signify the Scoliosis has been cured. Furthermore, if you give your sides a comfortable stretch frequently, you will improve the health of the inner organs and the blood circulation of your whole body.

(13) The Cat pose

Improves hormonal balance

1- Kneel down in the diamond pose, then bend forward and place both hands on the floor in front, keeping the weight transferred on your knees. Your hands should be shoulder distance apart, and your knees touching.

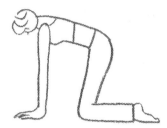

2- While breathing out, curve your back, look to the floor and bring in your stomach as you come to the end of the exhalation.

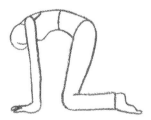

3- While breathing in, bend back and look up as far as you can as you end the inhalation.

Return to (2) while breathing out.

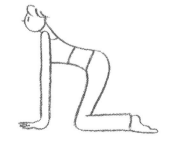

4- While breathing in, tilt your head up, bend back and bring your right leg up behind you.

Finish your inhalation once you have bent back sufficiently and hold your breath in this position for five seconds.

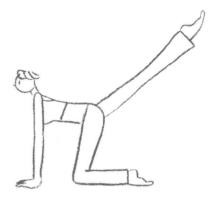

5- Return to (2) while breathing out.

6- Repeat (4), (5) with the left leg, then return to the diamond pose and breathe naturally. Repeat the pose one more time.

Relax in the Shava-asana pose

Notes:

Those who have a painful lower back should lift their leg up as far as it will go without hurting. This will ease the backache.

Be aware of your spine as you arch and curve your back and the balance of your hormones and function of your ovaries and womb will improve as a result. A woman I knew who had been worrying about irregular periods and not being able to conceive started to practise various poses where the legs are separated, concentrating mainly on the Cat pose. After ten months, her periods became regular again, and two years later she gave birth.

Now practise the Sun Worship pose (p.17) followed by the Leg Ki exercises (1 to 4) (p.73-80). After you have gathered Ki with the Leg Ki exercises, continue with the following 'Bending to the side with legs astride' pose.

(14) Bending to the side with legs astride pose

Strengthens the lumber region by stimulating the lumber vertebrae

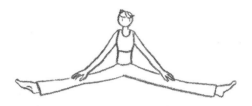

1- Sit down with your legs straight in front of you.

2- Stretch each leg out to the side as far as you can.
Push on the knees with your hands to ensure they do not leave the floor.

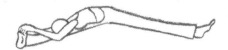

3- Clasp the big toe of your right foot with you right hand, turn your upper body to the right, and place your left hand on top of your right hand. While breathing out, lower your body to the right as far as you can until the end of the exhalation, then breathe naturally. Feel the stretch in the tendons of your feet.

4- While breathing in, bring your body up silently, release your hands, and face forwards again.
Do the same for your left side.

(15) *Bending forward with legs astride pose*

Practise after the 'Bending to the side with legs astride' pose

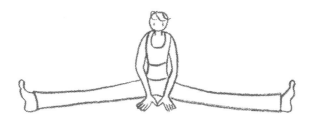

1- Spread your legs open wide and place your hands in the space in front. While breathing in, tilt your head upwards, stretching your back until the end of the inhalation.

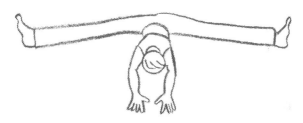

2- Breathe out, sliding your hands forward and lowering your body towards the floor. Finish the inhalation when you have gone as far as you can, then breathe naturally, keeping this pose. If you stop breathing here your muscles will stiffen and the pain you feel will be amplified, so focus on your exhalations. As your muscles relax, the pain will recede. Eventually, as you master the pose, you will be able to lower your forehead, chest and stomach onto the floor in front.

3- While breathing in, raise your body up silently and breathe naturally.

(16) Bending forwards while joining the soles of the feet together pose

Practise after the 'Bending forwards with legs astride' pose

1- Sit with your legs together in front and bend them so that the soles of the feet are together. Hold your ankles and bring the legs up to the torso.

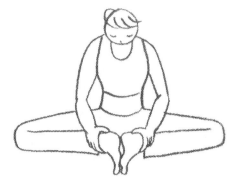

2- While breathing in, open your chest out and straighten your back.

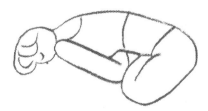

3- While breathing out, bend forwards as far as you can, then breathe naturally. As you become proficient at this pose you will be able to bend down so that your chin is on the floor. Each time you breathe out, make yourself go down further and eventually you will be able to lower the chest flat onto the floor.

4- While breathing in, bring your body up silently then breathe naturally.

Relax in the Shava-asana pose

Notes:

In poses 14, 15 and 16, keep your back straight since this will stimulate your groin muscles and correct any misalignments in your spine.

It will also cure sciatica and prevent hernias.

Please make sure your knees stay flat on the floor when you stretch the legs even if this means you can only bend forwards a small amount. You will not get the benefits of the pose if you let them rise up.

As you bend down, lead with the chest. Leading with the face will cause the back to become round. At first you may not be able to bend down far, but with practise you will eventually be able to lower your chest onto the floor.

This pose stimulates the lympa glands in the joints of the leg, which improves the balance of the hormones and function of the womb and ovaries. It is thus a particularly useful pose for women to practise.

(17) The Reverse pose

Stimulates the neck and shoulders, and encourages blood flow

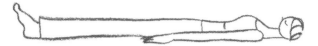

1- Sit down on the floor with your legs together in front and lie down face up. Place your arms alongside your body with your palms on the floor.

2- Breathe in and bring your legs up while keeping them straight, ending the inhalation when they are perpendicular to the floor.

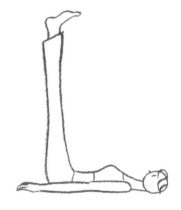

3- While breathing out, push on your palms and lift your lower back up off the floor then breathe naturally in this position. Your body should resemble the Japanese character ' く ' ('Ku'). Hold this pose for a short while.

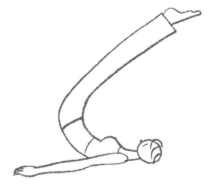

(18) Shoulder balancing pose

Follows from the Reverse pose

1- While in the '‹' position, put both hands on the lower back, then breathe out, raising both lower back and legs until they are in a straight line perpendicular to the floor. End your exhalation at this point then breathe naturally.

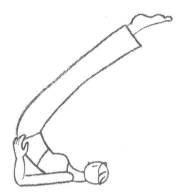

2- Keep your breathing regulated and silent, and hold this pose for twenty seconds to thirty seconds. Press your chin against the dip in your throat and concentrate on this point.

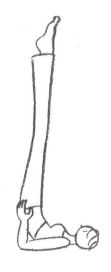

(19) The Plough pose

Follows from the Shoulder balancing pose

1- While breathing out, silently bend your legs down to the space above your head and finish the inhalation when your toes reach the floor. Breathe naturally in this position. If your toes do not yet reach the floor easily do not force them to.

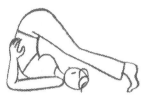

2- Release your hands from your lower back and clasp your hands on the floor underneath your back, interlocking the fingers. If you are able to, twist the wrists up, as this will stimulate the elbows and shoulders. The pressure on the throat in this pose will be more acute than in the Shoulder balancing pose.

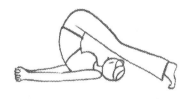

3- Relax the wrist back down and move the hands towards the head. For those flexible enough, clasp your toes. Maintain this pose for a while.

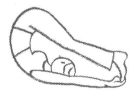

4- Release your hands from your toes and move them to the area below the back, keeping your palms flat on the floor.

5- While breathing out, lift your legs to a forty five degree position and breathe naturally.

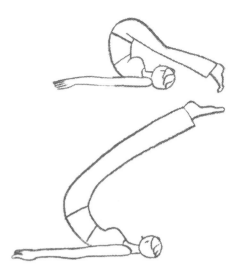

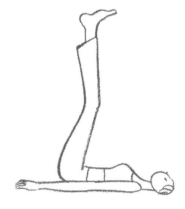

6- While breathing out, lower your back onto the floor. Finish the exhalation when the lower back reaches the floor, then breathe naturally.

7- While breathing out, lower your legs to the floor. Finish the exhalation when they reach the floor, then breathe naturally.

Relax in the Shava-asana pose

Notes:

In this pose, a considerable amount of pressure is put on the neck and shoulders, so it is important not to force yourself to do a movement when you feel resistance. If you do, there is a danger you may damage the cervical vertebrae.

This pose is effective in reducing stiffness and promoting blood flow in the neck and shoulders.

(20) Standing on the head pose (Headstand)

Reduces swelling and clears the head

1- From the diamond pose, sit up on your toes.

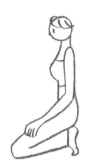

2- Bend your upper body forwards with clasped hands, move them onto the floor in front so your hands and elbows are on the floor. Make sure your elbows are separated shoulder width. If they are wider than this, it may not be stable enough to support the pose.

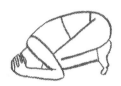

3- Lower your head so that the back part of the head is against your palms and the crown of the head (where a tsubo point is located) is touching the floor.

4- Stretch your knees and straighten your legs, pushing your bottom into the air. Move your toes nearer to your face and gradually make your upper body perpendicular to the floor.

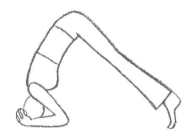

5- As you bring your thighs closer to your stomach, your upper body acts as a counter weight to your legs, which will start coming up automatically off the floor.

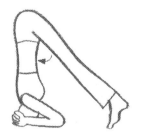

6- While keeping your balance, lift your legs up and bend your knees.

7- Breathe in and while keeping your knees bent, bring your legs up further until your thighs are perpendicular to the floor. Finish your inhalation at this point.

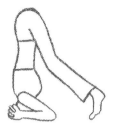

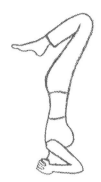

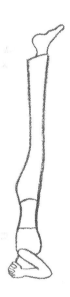

8- While breathing out, extend your knees and toes upwards. Finish your exhalation and continue breathing naturally when your legs and body are straight. Breathe silently and rhythmically as you keep this pose for a short while.

9- While breathing out, gradually bring your legs down again in the opposite order you raised them up, returning to (3).

10- Place your fists on top of each other on the floor and rest your forehead on them. Rest in this position for the same time as you balanced on the head in the pose.

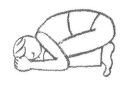

Relax in the Shava-asana pose

Notes:

When doing this headstand pose you may find the tendency to move the position of your head forward in order to prevent yourself from falling. However, moving the head towards the forehead has the effect of hurting the neck and shoulders. Make sure, therefore, that your head is resting on the crown before starting this pose. Simple adjustment of the position of your head will make any pain disappear.

For those who have pain in their eyes, ears or nose, have high blood pressure, are in their menstruation period, or are either suffering from an illness or have just recovered from one, please refrain from doing this pose.

For those who are too fearful to do the headstand, please practise steps (1) to (4).

Those who are unable to do the pose by themselves can make it safer by using a wall. Keep an appropriate space between the head and the wall. Be careful- make it too wide and you may hit your lower back hard against the wall if you lose balance.

It is also possible to get someone to hold your legs from the side. The person should just place his/her hands lightly on your legs and release occasionally in order for you to learn how to achieve balance by yourself.

Column 4

The 'father' of the poses

This 'standing on the head' pose is named the 'father of the poses' as it is one of the most advanced and important poses in Yoga. (For interest's sake the 'mother' of the poses is the 'standing on the shoulders' pose).

As you will know if you have practised it, the pose enables fresh blood to surge into the head, making your head feel light and refreshed. Also, when you return to your normal position after the pose, all impurities and blockages are released and exit the body together.

In this pose, the organs are all considerably stimulated as they are lifted up. You can also tell that your blood circulation has improved by the buzzing in your hands and feet after your finish the pose. From an aesthetic standpoint too, it will work in reducing swelling in the face so that the face appears smaller, and the eyelids more pronounced. It is because of these distinct effects that this pose is called 'the father' of the poses.

When you finish all twenty poses, practise the Single nostril breathing exercise A and B, the Re-energizing breathing exercise, the Depression alleviating breathing exercise, the Refreshing breathing exercise, and the Brain breathing exercise for insomnia (p.103) before relaxing in the Shava-asana pose.

At the end of my Yoga class, when everyone is relaxing in the Shava-asana pose, I say aloud the following words. You can say the words in your mind while you are relaxing.

Words spoken to your body

My right foot is relaxed. My right ankle is relaxed. My right calf is relaxed. My right knee is relaxed. My right thigh is relaxed. My right leg is relaxed. All the tension is now released from my right leg.

Repeat the same for the left leg.

My intestines are relaxed. My stomach is relaxed. My heart is relaxed. My lungs are relaxed. My neck is relaxed.

The fingers of my right hand are relaxed. My right wrist is relaxed. My right elbow is relaxed. My right shoulder is relaxed. My right arm is relaxed. All the tension is now released from my right arm.

Repeat the same for the left arm.

My jaw is loosened. My teeth are aligned comfortably. My mouth is relaxed. My nose is relaxed. My ears are relaxed. My eyes are relaxed. My forehead is relaxed. My head is now relaxed.

My arms feel heavy. My arms are comfortably stuck to the floor. My back is comfortably stuck to the floor.

My legs feel heavy. My legs are comfortably stuck to the floor.

My whole body is very comfortably stuck to the floor.

My mind and body is now completely relaxed.

Now take time to fully relax in the Shava-asana pose.

After seven to ten minutes of relaxing in the pose, open your eyes gently, and move your hands and feet slowly, signalling to the body that you are about to get up. When you have regained your strength and your mind is active again, slowly get up.

Lesson Four

Kikō

The key to Kikō

Kikō (Qigong) is the training and discipline of Ki. It is said that in China, there are as many as three thousand schools of Kikō. Ki is a specific type of energy which circulates the body. Improving this circulation through cultivating Ki can help overcome illnesses and when Ki is cultivated daily, an amazing state of health can be achieved.

The key to Kikō is the same as for Yoga, which is to make movements while removing all tension from the mind and body.

There are those who may say they don't know how to feel the presence of Ki, but anyone who is alive and breathing has Ki and is able to generate it. It is especially strong after practising Yoga, Kikō, or breathing exercises.

When you first start practising Kikō, you will experience Ki as a strange, warm, expansive sensation. The more you practise Kikō, the more this sensation will turn into something more definite and tangible.

Exercise Schedule

Dōkō is the practice of slow and steady movements to feel the physical presence of Ki flow in the body.

The basic practises of Dōkō is bringing Ki up and down, and opening up a Ki space from left to right. By practising these exercises, your sensation of Ki will become sharper.

Once you become proficient at both the vertical and horizontal Ki exercises, you can start to practise dropping Ki from your chest down to your tanden region.

There is a trick to dropping Ki from your chest to your tanden region. When you hold your breath after breathing in, contract your sphincter muscles at the same time and relax them as you breathe out. By doing so, you will be able to feel the Ki dropping from your chest to your abdomen. When contracting the sphincter muscles, don't be forceful. This is something which will become easier the more you practise.

These simple Leg Ki exercises are able to balance the mind and body in a short space of time. Practising them in between poses will make you more sensitive to the flow of Ki in the body.

Moving Ki up and down

1- Stand with your legs shoulder-width apart.

2- With palms facing upwards, raise your arms up the front of your body and imagine the Ki inside your body rising up from your feet to your head.

3- Turn your palms face down and lower them down the front of your body. As you do so imagine Ki flowing down from your head to your feet.

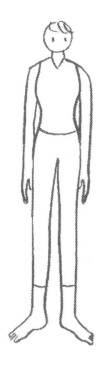

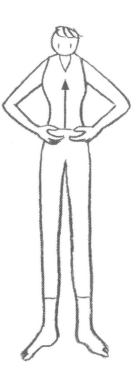

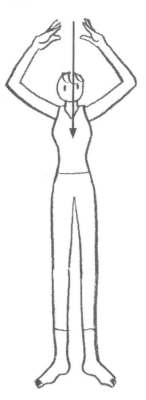

Creating Ki in a horizontal space

1- Imagine holding a ball of Ki.

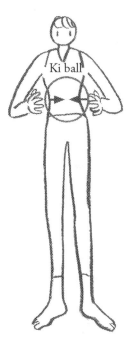

2- Get a feeling of the Ki by bringing your palms back and forth from each other.

When you bring your hands away from each other, imagine the ball of Ki expanding. When you bring your hands closer together imagine the ball shrinking in size.

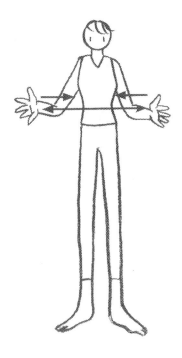

Notes:

The key to Dōkō is the same as for Yoga, which is to practise the movements when the mind and body are relaxed. To relax your muscles, you must be able to detect where the tension is and make it disappear as if switching off a light. In order to do this you must be able to move the body without using excess tension.

All of us move without thinking and so are mostly unaware of how much tension we have in the body.

When you start being mindful of your body's movements, you will notice that you are putting an unnecessary amount of tension in the body.

This could be when you are balancing yourself with the hanging strap in a train, or writing in a notebook. Also, when driving alone for the first time after passing your driving test, one normally tires from over-tensing the shoulders.

The way to remedy this is to be aware of your body. If you find you are using an unnecessary amount of tension, work out what the minimum amount of tension you need is and release the excess tension accordingly.

If you repeat this many times your body will remember not to overexert itself and you will gradually be able to stop becoming tense.

Column 5

The root of Ki

The first historical use of the character 'Ki' (気) dates back to the Shunjū period of warring states around two thousand seven hundred years ago.

A passage was made through the snowy peaks of the Himalyas linking India to China and enabling Indian medicine and Buddhism to enter China. It is believed that initially Prana (life energy, breathing and spiritual power), which was a part of the medicinal science of Yoga, was translated as '風' ('kaze,' meaning 'wind') before becoming '気.' ('The Health science of Ki, Meditation and Yoga,' Hiroshi Motoyama, Meicho kankōkai publishers).

As in India, Taoist masters in China were also said to have felt Prana energy in their practices. I imagine these Taoist masters experienced the same warm and comforting feeling of Prana as I do when practising Yoga.

The character for Ki, '気' is a simplified version of the original character '氣.'

It is made up of the characters '米' and '气,' giving it the literal meaning 'the steam from boiling rice.' It seems logical to me that the Taoist masters constructed this character for Prana with its warm and comforting effect in mind.

The next Dōkō exercise has been integrated into Prana Yoga from the ancient 'Daishūten' and 'Leg breathing' exercises and is called the 'Leg Ki exercise.' When practised inbetween Yoga poses, sensitivity to Ki can be increased.

Leg Ki exercise 1

1- Stand with your legs shoulder width apart. Relax your neck and shoulders. Let the mind gather around the abdomen; it will naturally when the upper body and especially the shoulders are relaxed. When the weight of your body centres around the abdomen your lower body will feel heavy and your feet will feel fixed to the floor.

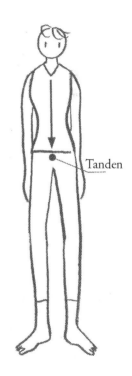

Tanden

2- Now imagine breathing in from both the top of your head (the Hyakue tsubo) and from the soles of your feet (the Yūsen tsubo). The Ki from the heavens and the Ki from the earth will meet at the abdomen. Hold your breath and imagine this Ki converging together. Now exhale this mixture of Ki through the soles of your feet.

Repeat this three times.

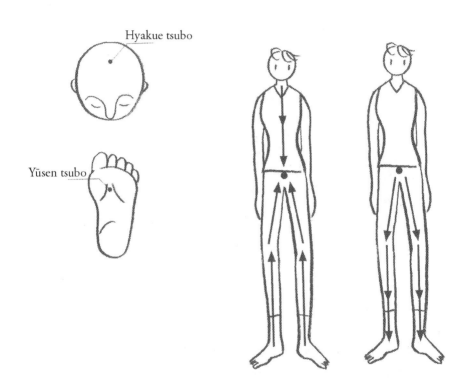

Hyakue tsubo

Yūsen tsubo

Leg Ki exercise 2

1- Without using your hands, imagine breathing in from the soles of your feet.

Next, draw the Ki up by concentrating on the soles of your feet, then your ankles, your calves, knees, thighs, abdomen, chest, throat, face and the crown of your head. (When bringing up Ki from your throat to your face, keep your tongue against the top of your mouth).

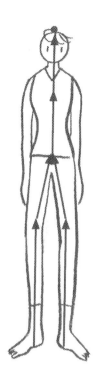

2- Hold your breath and keep concentrating on the crown of your head, then drop the Ki to your tanden.
(The trick to dropping Ki down to your tanden is to do it while holding your breath. If you try and drop Ki whilst exhaling it will stay in the head and not go down).

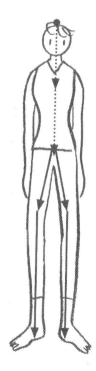

3- Once you have dropped Ki down to your tanden, exhale and expel the Ki down through your legs and out the soles of your feet.

Repeat this three times.

Leg Ki exercise 3

1- This exercise is the same as Leg Ki exercise 2 but with movements.

While breathing out, bend your upper body but leave your arms hanging down in front of you.

Draw a breath from the soles of your feet, as in exercise two, and when your fingers are lightly touching the floor, draw the Ki up to the crown of your head and raise your arms into the air.

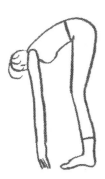

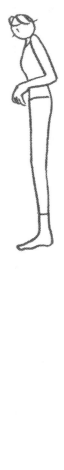

2- When you have drawn the Ki up to the crown of your head, hold your breath, and drop the Ki to your tanden.

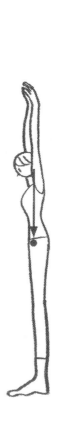

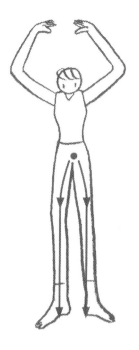 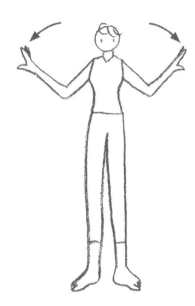

3- Turn your palms outwards, then exhale from the tanden out through the soles of your feet, bringing your arms down in an arc-shape as you do so.

When you bring your arms down, you should feel a radiant warm, tingling sensation which tells that your sensitivity to Ki has been activated.

Repeat this three times.

Leg Ki exercise 4

1- Breathe in from the soles of your feet and draw the Ki up to the crown of your head as in Leg Ki exercise 2.

Turn your palms so they are facing upwards, bend the elbows and bring your arms up to chest height.

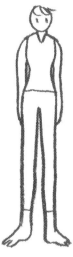

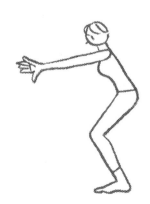

2- Hold your breath, drop the Ki from your head to your tanden. As you exhale through the soles of your feet, bend your knees and hold your arms outstretched in front of you with the top of your hands touching each other and little fingers directed upwards.

3- Inhale from the soles of the feet, release your hands from each other in an arc-movement, bringing them over your head. The palms should now be over your head and facing outwards.

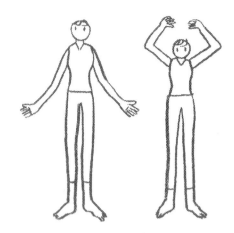

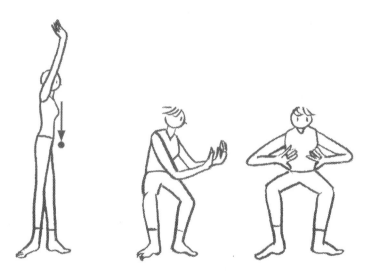

4- Hold your breath, drop the Ki from your head to your tanden, turn your upper body to the left then, while exhaling through the soles of your feet, bend your knees and face forwards.

5- Breathe in from the soles of your feet, make an arc with your arms, straighten your knees and draw the Ki up to the crown of your head as in (3).

As in (4), hold your breath and drop the Ki down to the tanden, turning your upper body this time to the right.

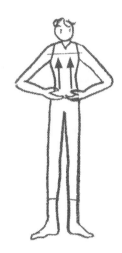

6- Again, as in (4), bend your knees and face forwards.
Breathe in from the soles of your feet and while straightening your knees, turn your palms so they are facing upwards and bring them up to a height level to your chest while drawing the Ki to the crown of your head.

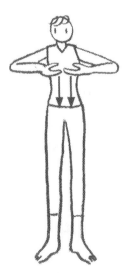

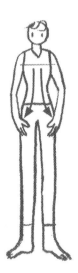

7- Hold your breath and drop the Ki to your tanden. Breathe out and drop the Ki to the soles of your feet while lowering your hands to your side.

Repeat this twice.

Column 6

The power of your little finger

In the body are pathways where Ki circulates. These pathways are called 'Keiraku' (meridians). The 'Kei' part of the word means 'vertical' and signifies the thick channels of Ki that run vertically in the body. The 'Raku' part of the word means 'to entwine' and signifies the thin channels of Ki that run across the body.

There are in total forty-four channels of Ki, running either horizontally or vertically in the body. Out of these are twelve main Keiraku.

According to Chinese teachings of Keiraku, all fingers and thumbs correspond to different parts of the body. The thumb is connected to the lungs via the lung meridian, the index finger is connected to the large intestines via the large intestine meridian, the middle finger is connected to the area around the heart via the pericardium meridian, the third finger is connected to the Sanjiao meridian which controls the 'three heats' (the heat produced from breathing, eating and excreting) and finally the little finger is connected to the heart via the heart meridian.

The little finger is capable of amazing things. To demonstrate this, here is something you can try for yourself.

First, stand as you would normally. Get someone to push your lower back gently from behind so that your body falls forward.

Now bend your little finger and concentrate on it. Strangely enough, this time when you are pushed from behind you will not budge an inch. No doubt for this reason, in the Japanese Martial Art of Kendo, all fingers clasped around the bamboo sword are relaxed except for the little finger which is tensed. I believe it is the same for Golf.

In this way, harnessing the power of the little finger can yield surprising results.

How to Collect Ki

Sensing and collecting the Ki that circulates the body

1- When the palms are brought closer together you should feel a strangely radiant and tingling sensation of Ki.
Now make a warm ball of Ki with your hands.

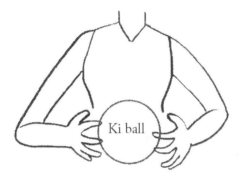

2- Place the Ki ball on the Hyakue tsubo (on the crown of your head). It should feel warm.

Move the Ki ball up and down so that you sense it against your head.

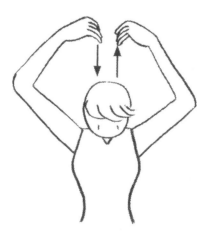

3- Now cover your forehead with both hands. It should feel warm and radiant. Do the same for your throat, chest, and solar plexus.

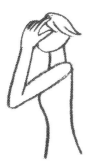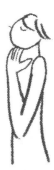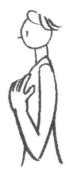

4- Cover your tanden with your hands. You should be able to sense this area (5cm below the belly button) particularly strongly.

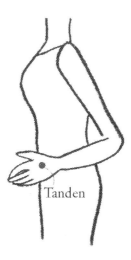

Tanden

5- As you move your palms towards and away from your tanden, you should feel a strange sensation of pressure, as if the Ki from your abdomen is repelling the Ki from your hands.

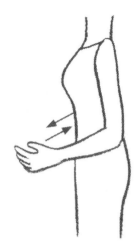

6- Place your hands on your tanden, transferring the Ki inside.

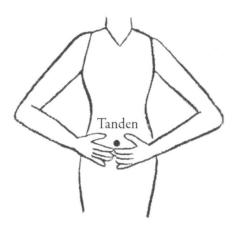

Tanden

Questions on Ki therapy

Q: If you can create Ki, does that mean you can heal people?

A: Yes it does. It seems for some people it is a difficult thing to believe in, as I often get asked by people if it is actually possible to heal with Ki. If you think about it though, it is something that all of us have experienced at some point. If, for example, someone complains of a painful stomach, the most natural thing to do is to put your hand on the person's stomach. Nobody would think of placing their hand on the person's head. I remember a time when I was young I was crying because I had hit my leg and my mother rubbed the painful area with her palm, saying 'pain, pain, go away.' Curiously enough it normally did go away. I believe this was because Ki was being emitted from her palms.

There are two types of Ki: Internal Ki and External Ki. Internal Ki is when the Ki is inside the body. Therapeutic and Remedial Ki therapy works in strengthening the Internal Ki, with the aim of increasing health and curing illnesses.

External Ki on the other hand, is when the Internal Ki exits the body and forms externally. Only Ki therapists who have undertaken extensive Ki training will be able to produce this type of Ki.

Q: What are the methods of using this External Ki?

A: These are the following methods for using External Ki.

1- Placing a hand on the area.

2- Putting the hand above the area (covering technique).

3- Emitting Ki from the area inbetween the eyebrows (the Ajna Chakra, for example)

4- Practise Ki from image creation only (prayer and remote therapy).

Out of these, only (1) and (2) is possible for anyone to do (although there are, of course, discrepancies in strength).

However, one thing to bear in mind is that if an untrained person tries to copy what a Ki therapist does and uses their own energy in applying Ki, they will feel completely exhausted afterwards.

Q: How does someone emit Ki effectively without causing harm to themselves?

A: Since the External Ki technique can be tiring on the body, it is safer for an ordinary person to use the unlimited source of Ki in the universe.

To do this, imagine the unlimited Ki of the universe entering the body via the Hyakue tsubo and flowing from your hand into the affected part of the person you are treating.

As this is happening, remove all feelings of wanting to heal the person from your mind. If you have those feelings, you will use your own energy and end up extremely tired. Try and practise Ki on a member of your family who has pain somewhere on their body. If Ki is transferred successfully, the pain will either go down or disappear.

Beware though; if you try and practise on someone who is very ill, their negative Ki may be stronger than your own Ki, creating an imbalance and making you ill as a result. As long as they are a family member it should be fine.

Column 7

The secret of Ki therapy is releasing tension from the body

I first realised the amazing power that comes from releasing tension from the body when I treated a businessman for a sprained back.

The man was suffering from extreme pain in his lumber region. He was unable even to turn at night, and had already taken two weeks off work. His wife had phoned me up at night telling me he was completely immobile and begged for my help. When I went around to their house at night, the man told me that he always got a sprained back every four years, 'just like the Olympics' he joked, but added, 'this time has been the most painful up till now.'

After the first session, he was able to turn again at night. After the second session he was able to stand, and after the third session, he was finally able to walk to the toilet.

The following day, a golf competition was held in which employees of the major Japanese companies in the UK competed against each other.

The man was an employee of one of these companies and was extremely grateful just to be able to take part in such a well-known competition after only recently suffering from a sprained back.

Since his sprained back had been so painful he played very tentatively, making sure he released all the tension in his body for each swing. I say making sure, but he didn't have a choice; he was unable to put tension in his shoulders and other parts of his body without hurting his back.

By playing in this way, the man ended up winning the whole competition. No one was more surprised than the man himself. The competition was known far and wide, and the other competitors were businessmen who had trained extensively so that they might be able to claim the much coveted title as their own.

What happened to this man is a vivid example of the amazing power that removing tension from the body brings.

Afterwards, people apparently disputed his victory, suggesting that in the two weeks he had taken off work for his sprained back he was actually practising intensively for the competition. When he received the trophy therefore, he made sure he mentioned the Ki treatment as the reason for his swift recovery.

The following day, my phone rang continuously with calls from people who were keen on undertaking treatment to improve their golf. In no way can I guarantee that Ki therapy will improve one's proficiency at golf and for that reason I duly refused all requests.

Lesson Five

Breathing Exercises
Yoga breathing exercises to re-invigorate the mind and body

In India, breathing exercises were developed to deepen meditation and thus increase one's level of spiritual attainment.

Controlling the breath trains the ability to control the autonomic nerve enabling a spiritual level of relaxation. I for one can say with certainty that a deeper level of meditation can be achieved after practising Yoga.

On the other hand, in China, more of the focus was on physical practicality. Ki and breathing developed into a myriad of techniques, with applications for Martial Arts, health benefits and medicinal treatment.

In Yoga, breathing exercises are called Pranayama. Controlling Prana or Ki (life energy) is called the 'Chōki' method in Japanese.

Breathing exercises in Yoga are not merely for taking in oxygen. They are also used to deepen meditation and bring into the body the energy that fills the cosmos.

The Key to Breathing Exercises

In Yoga, the nose is used for breathing, and except for special cases, the mouth is not. Through practice, one can get used to breathing like this at all times. Although this may seem a trivial matter, it is actually very important.

When you breathe from your nose, the nose hairs trap the big dust particles in the air. The smaller dust particles are then trapped by the nasal membrane. The air is then warmed up by the nasal passage until it reaches a sufficient level of humidity before entering the lungs.

Breathing from the mouth, however, aggravates the throat and lungs by bringing in dust and cold, dry air. In many cases, young people get ill these days from breathing from their mouths.

Some breathing exercises also have the effect of stimulating and reactivating the brain.

Yoga, in particular, has a number of breathing exercises where breathing is switched between the right and left nasal passages.

Breathing slowly through a single nostril stimulates the nerves that control the sense of smell. These nerves are directly connected to the brain which is invigorated as a result.

For this reason, breathing exercises can act in preventing dementia in elderly people. Apparently the disease is rare among practitioners of 'Kōdō' (the Japanese art of appreciating incense) which again, must be due to the fact that the brain is invigorated when the nerves controlling the sense of smell are stimulated.

Also, continued practice of Yoga breathing exercises will make you feel energetic and alive. This is because using the stomach diaphragm when you breathe in enables your lungs to fill with oxygen. When breathing using the diaphragm, the forty six square metres used by the lungs increases twofold to ninety two square metres.

As the lungs fill up with oxygen, it is in turn delivered to all six trillion cells which make up the body, creating a healthy structure resistant to illnesses including cancer.

Recently the medical world has realised this fact and are beginning to recommend breathing exercises as a way of strengthening the immune system and defending the body against disease.

Sitting when doing breathing exercises is either in the Lotus (Padma-āsana) or Half-Lotus (Siddha-āsana) poses or if this is not possible, on a chair. However way you sit, it must be with a straight back. Join your index fingers and thumbs together in the 'Jnana-mudra' (symbol of wisdom).

In breathing exercises, normally only the right hand is used, except in special cases. This comes from the culture in India where the right hand is always clean and used for eating, while the left hand is dirty and used for when going to the toilet. There are many effects depending on which breathing exercise you practise, so pick ones which are suitable for your body and state of health.

Lotus pose

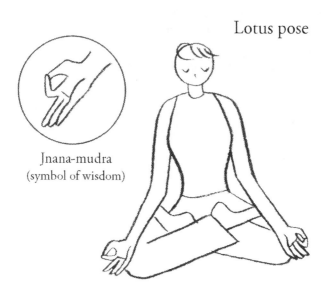

Jnana-mudra
(symbol of wisdom)

Half-Lotus pose

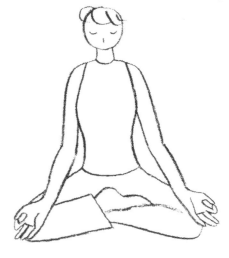

Single nostril breathing exercise A (Anuloma Viloma A)

1- With your elbow at shoulder height, press all of your fingers (except the thumb) of your right hand on your left nostril and breathe in from the right nostril. Exhale all the air out of the right nostril in one burst.

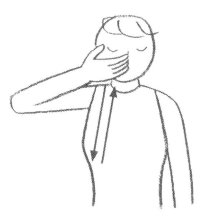

2- After exhaling, press your thumb on your right nostril and breathe in from the left nostril. Exhale all the air out of the left nostril in one burst.

Repeat this ten times for both nostrils.

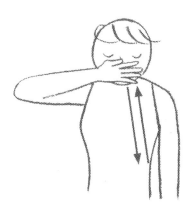

Single nostril breathing exercise B (Anuloma Viloma B)

1- Press your right nostril with your right thumb and breathe in from your left nostril. Immediately hold the left nostril and expel all the air out of your right nostril in one burst.

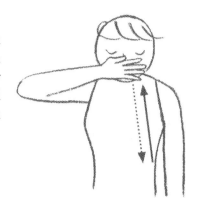

2- Immediately after breathing out, breathe in from the right nostril then hold the right nostril and expel the air out of the left nostril. Now breathe in from the left nostril and expel the air out of the right nostril, then breathe in from the right nostril and expel the air out of the left nostril and so on in this pattern, rhythmically breathing in immediately after breathing out.

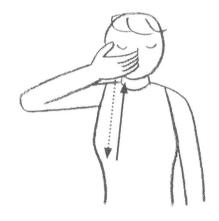

Notes:

These breathing exercises remove impurities in the nose enabling breathing to become smooth. People are known to have cured their hayfever with these breathing exercises.

Re-energizing breathing exercise (*Agni Prasārana*)

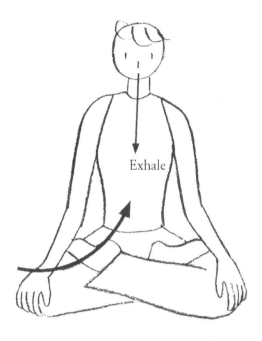

1- Rest your hands on top of your knees. Inhale, bringing in your stomach and exhale sharply through both nostrils.

2- Immediately after exhaling, breathe in then exhale again sharply through both nostrils, drawing in your stomach as you do so. In this breathing exercise, the diaphragm will move up and down as the breath is exhaled and the stomach is drawn in.

Practise this fifty times in a row.

Notes:

This re-energizing breathing exercise is very powerful, so if you find yourself getting light-headed, practise it just ten times at the beginning and build up gradually from there. Drawing in the stomach seems easy but is in fact quite a tricky thing to do. It is therefore necessary to practise it a number of times to get the hang of it.

The state of the mind is shown in the organs. A person who has a hard and cold stomach will not have much vigour. Once the stomach starts to move, however, he or she will start to retain vigour.

If you are someone who is always tense, on edge and unable to relax, feel your solar plexus. Is it hard? Push into the centre with your fingertip. Pain will signify that you are under stress or that your stomach is tired. Now press into the central edge of your ribs on the right side of your body. If it is painful it means you often get angry about things. If this is the case for you, then this breathing exercise will be particularly effective. By practising this breathing exercise, the solar plexus will be massaged and the hardness will dissipate. The breathing will then deepen and you will find you are able to relax.

Depression alleviating breathing exercise (Nādi Shodhan)

1- Raise your right elbow up to shoulder height and bend your index finger and middle finger. Press your left nostril with the outstretched third finger and little finger and breathe steadily and silently through your right nostril.

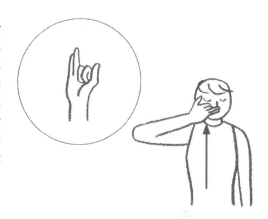

2- When you have finished breathing in, press your right nostril with your thumb and breathe slowly out of your left nostril.
When you have finished breathing out, breathe in from your left nostril.

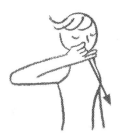

3- Hold your left nostril and breathe slowly out of your right nostril. Your exhalation should be twice as long as your inhalation.

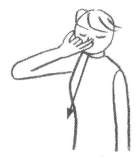

Notes:

It is important with this breathing exercise to inhale and exhale silently. Count to five as you breathe in and count to ten as you breathe out. If this is too long for you, count to four as you breathe in and eight as you breathe out. As you get used to the breathing exercise you can lengthen your exhalation by increasing your count.

In Yoga, the right nostril leads to the Sun Ki channel (the Pingala) which is warm and enables the mind to look outward. The left nostril, on the other hand, leads to the Moon Ki channel (Ida), which is cold and enables the mind to look inward. This is why if the balance between the nostrils is skewed, the mind can become restless or depressed. Those who feel they can't settle down easily should try this exercise.

I have recommended this breathing exercise to those suffering from depression, including a student studying abroad, and people who all kept on saying 'I wish I was dead' throughout the day. After practising this exercise, all reported a lightness of spirit; an amazing change to how they had been before.

Refreshing breathing exercise (Dirgha Shwāsa Prashwāsa)

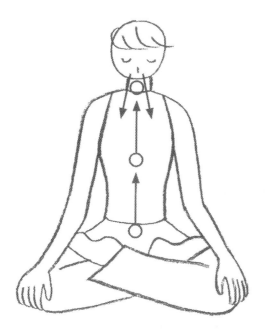

1- Place your hands on your knees. Breathe in strongly through both nostrils, filling your abdomen, chest, then your throat with air. Finish the exhalation when your throat is filled with air, hold your breath for a moment, then exhale strongly with both nostrils. Make a lot of sound with the exhalation.

2- Repeat this ten times.

Notes:

If ten times is too much you can start with a smaller number. This number can increase the more you practise Yoga and become accustomed to the breathing exercises.

The Refreshing Breathing Exercise clears the throat and lungs and frees the spinal Ki channel of blockages, leaving the person feeling refreshed and energized.

There was a youngster who enthused that practising the exercise for a hundred times in a row felt great and put him in a hazy state akin to inhaling strongly on a cigarette. I would, however, strongly advise against doing anything like this.

If a beginner practises a powerful breathing exercise over and over again, it can be harmful. There is also the possibility of loosening the cranium which can be very dangerous.

Cooling breathing exercise (Shītkārī)

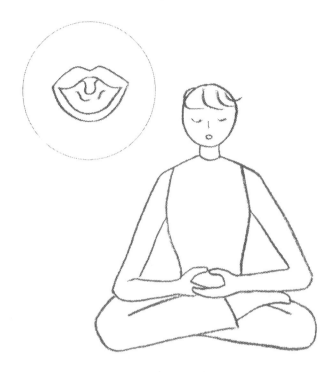

1- Join your hands in front, with fingers interlocked. Curl your tongue into a tube and inhale while making a sucking sound.

2- When you finish the inhalation, close your mouth and exhale immediately out of both nostrils.

Repeat this ten to twenty times.

Notes:

Since India is a hot country, there are many Yoga breathing exercises such as this one for cooling the body. However, while practising it in the summer is very useful, be careful practising it in the winter, especially if you have a cold constitution; it makes you get cold easily and can therefore have an adverse effect on the body.

I once knew a lady who, possibly because of menopausal reasons, had a hot upper body and felt dazed as a result. She discovered she liked this breathing exercise after trying it so she started practising it in succession. After practising it around twenty times, she measured her temperature and was delighted to see it had dropped two degrees. She therefore continued practising it for another five minutes. According to the woman, her temperature then dropped to a very low level causing her stomach to become painful and for her to feel very ill.

This shows the importance of practising the exercise only on days when it is hot and to stop when the body is at a comfortable temperature.

An added effect of this breathing exercise is to make the face appear more beautiful. When we do this exercise in my class, strangely enough, everyone, regardless of facial structure, appears beautiful.

Maybe noble is a better way of describing the face than beautiful. In any case, the face undergoes a spiritual transformation, and starts to resemble the face of the Buddha as depicted in the ancient images and statues. Every time I see this happen I am surprised and moved.

Brain breathing exercise for insomnia

1- Breathe in slowly, imagining the breath coming in from the crown of the head (the Hyakue tsubo).

2- Open the mouth slightly and exhale slowly and steadily. On this out breath, imagine all the waste matter and toxins in the body exiting from your mouth.

3- Breathe in from following tsubo in this order.

Zencho (5cm in front of the Hyakue tsubo) > Indō (centre of forehead) > Miken (between the eyebrows) > Taiyō (the temples) > Jinchū (space below the nose) > Amon (between the top two spinal vertebrae) > Gyokuchin (under the two protruding parts on the lower area of the skull).

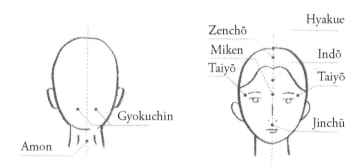

Notes:

This insomnia aiding brain breathing exercise is a simplified version of one of the exercises in the book 'Brain Breathing' (Lee Sung-hŏn and others, Business publishers).

It is an easy breathing exercise to do once you have remembered where all the various tsubo are on the head, and it has a surprisingly immediate effect: Just by practising it twice, your head will feel light and refreshed and you will be able to relax.

After practising it many times, you will get used to feeling the breath enter the brain from the tsubo as a narrow stream.

I recommended this exercise to someone suffering from insomnia and they told me that as a result, they were able to sleep well without the use of sleeping tablets and also that they felt good in the morning when getting up. (Taken from my book 'The Power of Life' from the passage 'Breathing Exercise for people who can't sleep at night').

Column 8

The Brain breathing exercise has the power to cure acute fatigue, pain and anxiety

I once knew a businessman who had a phobia of flying. Once, before a flight, as he started to get nervous his legs suddenly gave up on him at the gate in the airport. He phoned me, at a loss as what to do.

I advised him to sit on the nearest seat and practise the brain breathing exercise. He did so, and as a result, was able to check in without any problem. On the plane he practised the exercise again and fell into a deep sleep, even though normally he was unable to sleep at all. 'When I awoke I found I had already arrived at the destination,' he said, laughing.

Here is another story about someone who was invited to a dinner where he ate seafood. That night he had an excruciating pain in his stomach. He lay down on his bed, holding his stomach and wondered if he should take his stomach medicine. The thing was, whenever he took the stomach medicine, it always had an adverse effect on him which took weeks to recover from. That moment he suddenly remembered the brain breathing exercise so he sat on the corner of his bed and started practising it. By the time he had got to the Indō tsubo, (the third tsubo on the head) the pain had miraculously vanished from his stomach.

There are some people who cannot get over their fatigue even after a good night's sleep or a period of a couple months. These type of people would find the brain breathing exercise very useful. It is said that, in the case of physical fatigue, the chemicals in the blood that cause fatigue disappear in just an hour and a half of sleep. This shows that it therefore must be the brain, not the body which continues to feel tired. When sleeping does not relieve the feeling of fatigue, this brain breathing exercise will, by relieving the fatigue in the brain.

Lesson Six

Meditation Exercises

Why do Meditation?

It is said that the three main pillars of Yoga practice are Asanas (poses), Pranayama (Breathing Exercises) and Meditation.

When someone asks me why I do meditation, I tell them it is 'in order to remember our divine nature, our spiritual essence.'

Meditation is one method to re-discover the reason why we are existing here in this present moment by reminding ourselves of the soul. We practise meditation to re-awaken ourselves. Through meditation, we meet our true selves and understand that everything is one. This realisation leads to the understanding that all actions and happenings are part of the flow of the universe, a realisation that greatly changes how we look at the world and makes it possible to live in peace.

By doing meditation we can experience the sparkle of life in each moment within the flow of the universe.

There are not just one but many different methods of meditation. Meditation is not something you can do by thinking with the head. In fact it gets more difficult to do the more you try and analyse it. Here is a method of meditation which anyone can do and which requires no brain work.

The Key to Meditation

As you get used to meditation, you will able to do it anywhere. To start with, however, choose a room which is pleasant, quiet and free of distractions.

The best times to do meditation are in the morning and late afternoon or evening since at these times the wavelengths in the air are relaxing and good for meditation.

If you practise meditation in the morning, do it before breakfast and if in the late afternoon, before dinner. If you do it after dinner, make sure you wait at least two hours after eating. Doing it straight after dinner is detrimental to meditation, since blood accumulates around the stomach after a meal, reducing the amount of blood in the brain and making it hard to concentrate.

For daily meditation, I would recommend starting at five minutes, then gradually working your way up to twenty minutes, then to thirty minutes. As you get used to thirty minutes extend it up to an hour.

When sitting in meditation, keep a straight back. If you are able to, sit in the 'Lotus' (Padma-āsana) or 'Half Lotus' (Siddha-āsana) pose (p.92).

If your posture is bent forward while doing meditation it is hard to clear your mind of abstruse thoughts. Feel, therefore, as if your head is being pulled up gently. Place your hands gently on your lap, and join your index fingers and thumbs in 'Jnana-mudra' (p.92).

Normally the eyes are closed, but you can also practise meditation with them open. If you keep them closed, concentrate on either the middle of the eyebrows or the end of the nose and try not to move the eyeballs. If you keep your eyes open, look at the end of your nose or at a candle flame in order to keep your eyes still. Concentration is also lost if the tongue moves, so keep it fixed to the top of the mouth.

Yoga Meditation technique

1- Focus on a point.

All meditation techniques start by concentrating the mind on a fixed point (Gyōnen). Abstruse thoughts will come up, one after another, as when the mind is concentrating on a point, the power of the conscious mind is weakened, giving way to the stack of thoughts in the subconscious mind that had hitherto been suppressed.

2- Concentrate the mind on the middle of the eyebrows

Just watch the thoughts as they come up without trying to stop them and they will gradually reduce after a while. The key to this technique is not to try and stop the thoughts as they come up. Forcing it will have an adverse effect. Toy with the thoughts a little then return to concentrating on the middle of the eyebrows. Practise this meditation at the start for about five minutes everyday.

If you find this Yoga meditation technique difficult, here are three other meditation techniques; Mantra meditation, Breath counting and Mantra breathing meditation.

Notes:

When you concentrate in meditation, the breathing becomes extremely slow and rhythmical. You can tell whether or not you are in a state of meditation by checking your breathing. If it seems to have stopped or becomes very quiet and carries on like this for three to five minutes, then you have entered meditation.

Mantra Meditation technique

1- Make your own mantra.

This mantra can be made up of any words, as long as they make you feel good. In India 'Ohm' or 'Ohm Namah Shivaya' is used. In Tibetan Buddhism, 'Ohm Mani Padme Hum' and in Japan, positive words such as 'Peace,' 'Happiness,' 'Refreshing,' and 'Relaxing' are used.

2- When exhaling, recite the mantra in your mind. To start with, recite a short mantra to avoid running out of breath.

Try the mantra for a while to see if it suits you and change it if it doesn't. Do not worry about the breathing as it will naturally become ordered as you recite the mantra. At the start, practise for five minutes and increase this gradually to about twenty minutes.

Notes:

This is a meditation technique which is simple and easy enough for beginners to do but which can yield amazing results. I would recommend it for those who have not had much success with meditation before to try it.

It is possible to enter a deep state of meditation just by reciting a mantra. The meaning of mantra is 'true word.'

The key to practising the mantra technique is to approach it with child like innocence and recite the words with an empty mind.

You may find that while in meditation, your breathing becomes very still and you forget the words of the mantra. This has happened not because your technique is wrong, but because your meditation has become deeper. Just continue reciting the mantra once you start to think consciously again. When practising meditation, you will not be able to be in complete concentration from start to finish. You will have series of brief moments when the meditation is deep before it becomes shallow again. If you practise it daily, these deep moments will very slowly increase in length.

Counting your breaths

1- Chant 'one' in your mind as you exhale, then inhale.

2- Do the same for all the numbers up to ten.

3- Start again from one when you reach ten.

Notes:

This technique where the inhalation and the exhalation is used to count is called 'Ana Apana' in Sanskrit. As a part of Yoga it has been around in India since Ancient times, and has also been integrated into Buddhism and Ki therapy.

The technique consists of concentrating on the numbers and repeating the process many times. If you make a mistake in the number order, always start again from the beginning.

Mantra Breathing Meditation technique

1- Breathe in from the nose and say 'Hahn' in your mind.

2- While exhaling from the nose, say 'Sah' in your mind.

> Notes:
>
> This technique uses the Sanskrit mantra 'Hahn Sah' (or Horn Sor) which means 'I am he' (God). It is said that 'Hahn' and 'Sah' are derived from the vibrations of the inhalation and the exhalation which means that every time human beings breathe they are subconsciously reciting 'I am he (God)' which is the truth of our existence.
>
> The key to this technique is to concentrate on the breathing. When the concentration becomes strong enough, the breathing alone will be put you in a meditative state.
>
> In this sense it is the ultimate method of meditation.

Column 9

How to control the mind for spiritual concentration (Gyōnen)

As you begin to master the spiritual concentration you will be able to control the beginning and end of a thought.

One method to develop this is through intense practice of an extreme breathing exercise. (Note that this is not suitable for beginners). When the extreme breathing exercise is practised many times in succession, the mind becomes blank. Soon something will pop up on this blank canvas. As you watch this thing, it will occur to you that a thought is being born. As this thought starts to end it will disappear and a new thought will begin. As you observe this happening, you will start to feel a space between the end of one thought and the beginning of another. This space is where the mind is not working. Through practice it will gradually increase, enabling a backdrop of deep silence for the practitioner. As you immerse yourself in this feeling you will start to understand what the great philosopher Krishnamurti meant when he said, 'There is an expanding silence between one thought and another.'

Once you are able to do spiritual concentration well, change the object you are concentrating on. Imagine, for example, a glass of water and concentrate on the water inside. Imagine the water vividly, right down to the smallest detail, as if you are looking at a photo. Before long, your mind will become fixed on the water in the glass. This type of discipline, where something is imagined right down to the smallest detail, is called 'Gyōnen' in Japanese.

Once you can do this, start moving the glass of water around, and change the perspective of the container, as if you watching a recorded video of it. From above the cup, the water looks round. From the side, the water looks cylindrical. As you tip the glass horizontally, the water becomes a stream. As you drink the water, it passes the oesophagus, circles the organs, turns into urine and leaves the body.

In this way, the water, as the object of our concentration, is imagined in every scenario possible. This discipline is called 'Jōryo' in Japanese and is in fact Yoga meditation.

Finally, once you have explored in your imagination all the different scenarios which involve water, there ceases to be any difference between you and the water. In other words you become the water itself. This state is called 'Sanmai' in Japanese, the realm of enlightenment. 'Sanmai' is a discipline where you become one with the image you are concentrating on; the image itself becomes reality. The three practises of 'Gyōnen,' 'Jōryo' and 'Sanmai' are the most powerful of the image training exercises in Yoga.

Lesson Seven

Yoga in Daily Life

Simple contentment with Yoga

The Yoga Asanas I have covered in this book, will, if practised daily, have a considerable effect on your life.

Practising Yoga produces positive and peaceful waveforms in the mind which will attract only the things which are necessary to you. This will enable you to live a life of fulfillment; if something unpleasant happens, the positive waveforms in your mind will enable you to accept the situation calmly, learn an important lesson, and find the confidence to make a fresh new start.

I will now go over some important points for incorporating Yoga in your daily life.

1-Do not attempt to be perfect when doing Yoga

If you are only able to do Yoga once or twice a week, think of it as a great achievement. In time, you will see Yoga as something very pleasant to do, and you will start wanting to practise it more frequently. Before long you will want to practise it every day.

Since it is not usually so easy to make a good habit, think how fantastic it would be if you made a habit of doing Yoga.

2-Fix a time and place for doing Yoga

Save a period of time in the morning for doing Yoga. If you practise it at different times in the day it is hard to keep the practice up. If you keep a time fixed in the day, your body will become accustomed to the practice better and you will find it easier to continue.

Decide on where to practise. If you practise in the same place every time, the Ki energy which you emit will be absorbed in the walls and carpet, creating a personal 'Ki space.' Sitting in this Ki space will get you into the mood for practising Yoga.

3-Understand that relaxation is the real point of doing Yoga

After a pose in Yoga, lie down and relax. Do not forget that the relaxing is more important than the pose. Relaxation is indeed the whole point of Yoga.

When we relax and become one with the floor, we join with the universe. In so doing, we give way for the unlimited energy of the universe to recharge our body and mind. Relaxing not only makes us feel better but also gives us the strong realisation that the universe is making it possible for us to live.

If we are tense and cannot relax, therefore, this energy will not enter the body and we will become tired quickly. Stress will build up, causing damage to the body.

You can live in an ideal way by practising Yoga

When a person relaxes in Yoga, pleasant and bright waveforms are created which have the power to change one's life for the better and enable a person to live a life just as he/she envisages.

When waveforms are similar they attract each other, but when they are different they repel. Anxiety and fear, therefore, will attract similar negative energies.

In this way, those who constantly feel fear will be pulled into dangerous situations even if they reside in a safe place. I knew one person, for example, who lived in London, but had travelled to Kobe on the day the Kobe Earthquake happened and had a traumatic time as a result. There were also instances of people for whom the reverse happened.

Logically therefore, filling our minds with happy, peaceful and bright waveforms is something we should strive for. These waveforms will act on the outside world, turning our thoughts into reality. Remember- changing your own mind will change the world around you.

Furthermore, if you continue with Yoga, you will stop dwelling over trivialities and your attachment to things will decrease. As your mind gets filled with joy, you will become content with how you are living your life at the moment and will be filled with appreciation. You will become satisfied with the bare necessities in your daily life. Your life will become very simple, and enjoyably so.

As you delve even deeper into Yoga and meditation, the infinite energy of the universe will freely enter your body, enabling everything to go smoothly. When this happens, your dreams will become reality from the smallest effort and things which you would have thought were impossible will start to happen.

Creating reality through Meditation

Some time ago now I was desperate to go to India, and so made this a focus of meditation every day.

Normally, when someone plans on going to India, they would go to a tourist office which advertises sightseeing trips to India, and find out about the place they are going to by collecting information.

In order to find out about the best flight deals, they may go to various travel agencies to compare prices. I, however, did none of the above. I simply concentrated on meditation.

Every single day, as I meditated, I pictured an image of myself practising Yoga in the Himalayas.

At the break of dawn, cool Ki flows down into the meditation hall. I hear a rustling of leaves as a breeze blows through a grove. The breeze brings with it snippets of a unique birdsong. From where I am, I am able to look into a deep valley where the Ganges river meanders, shining and blue.

Everyday I pictured this in my mind during meditation.

Then after about two months, things started to happen.

First, the director of a travel agent company asked me for urgent treatment because he was worried his sprained back may prevent him from attending an important meeting the following day. By the end of the session he was so much better, he felt he was well enough to dance, and was very grateful for my help. When I told him about my wish to go to India, he mentioned that he had a spare agent discounted business class ticket from London to Bombay which had a reduction of seventy five percent off the original price. I therefore decided to buy it off him.

Next, I received a phone call from the wife of a businessman who had come back from working abroad and had cricked his neck while sleeping on the return flight.
She asked me to help him since he couldn't keep his head up straight. At the end of the session, this man too had made a full recovery and was able to hold his head straight again.

When I mentioned my trip to India, the couple told me that they had lived there for seven years due to the husband's work and could help me with anything I needed.

The following day they sent a Telex through to their best friend who was the head of the company's regional office in Bombay. They told me to ask him for advice on anything, even going so far as to write an introductory letter for me. The next day, the wife was cleaning the room and found a bundle of Indian rupee notes which she asked me to use in India, since the Indian currency hadn't much value in the UK.

I therefore enjoyed a comfortable trip in Business class on board a Canadian Airlines plane to Bombay, where I met the regional head of the business man's company as planned. The following day, he had arranged lunch for me with a group of experienced Yoga practitioners to whom I could find out all the information I wanted. The morning after that I went straight to the sacred grounds which are situated near the origin of the River Ganges in the Himalayas.

There, I stayed at a Hindu temple to practise meditation. At four in the morning I got up and sat in the meditation hall. Cool air flowed in. A breeze came and rustled the trees and carried with it wisps of a strange birdsong sung by a little bird.

As I looked down I saw the blue meandering Ganges river, blurred and glinting in the sun and realized I wasn't seeing it for the first time. This was the view I had pictured in my meditation in London. The image created in meditation had become one with reality, and had done so without any need for effort.

This method will not pass for an entrance exam, it must be said. No matter how much you time you put in imagining yourself celebrating passing your exam, if you don't do the relevant work, you will without doubt fail. This is the kind of situation where effort is needed to for a wish to become real.

Having said that, there are holy men in India who may disagree. There have been strange cases of people who had suddenly had an idea of what was going to come up in the exam the day before without studying for it, or had chanced upon an answer sheet on the ground when going for a walk, enabling them to pass the exam and graduate from University.

However, the fact remains that normal people such as ourselves must be content with doing the necessary work.

Column 10

With Meditation, doubt turns into conviction

If you practise meditation, eventually all preference and attachment to things on a deeper level of consciousness will disappear, enabling you to feel at one with the universe. When this happens, doubt in the mind will turn into four types of conviction or realisation.

The first type of realisation is when worldly mind changes and enters a state where it becomes a mirror and directly reflects the true state of the universe. This realisation is called 'Daien Kyōchi' in Japanese, or 'Great Mirror Wisdom.'

The second type of realisation is when, after the mind's attachment to the world disappears, all attachment to the self also disappears and other people, the self and nature all become one equal entity, a firm realisation born not in the head but in the deep recesses of the mind. This is called 'Byōdō Shōchi' in Japanese, or 'Awareness of equanimity wisdom.'

As the deep level of consciousness changes in this way, the conscious mind gains the wisdom to continually view the outside world as magnificent. This is the third type of realisation and is called 'Myōkan Zatchi' in Japanese or 'Wondrous intuition wisdom.'

Once a businessman came for therapy at my house during spring. In the garden the daffodils had flowered and the cherry blossoms were in full bloom. As I remarked how beautiful the cherry blossoms were, the man was very surprised, as he simply had not noticed them. People like this have become too attached to the workings of the self to observe the world around them.

When the conscious mind changes, the workings of the five senses begin to change also. With this realisation, the person will do the most necessary thing at any given time, like a housewife who sees a dirty table and decides to clean it immediately while she has time. This is the fourth realisation and is called 'Jōsho Sachi' in Japanese or 'Accomplishment Wisdom.'

In this way, if you continue with meditation, even if you may not achieve enlightenment, your doubts will gradually be replaced by understanding. We are all able to come to the realisation that we are part of the universe; we were born there to spend a short time in this life, and we will once again return back there. If deep down you can appreciate life and live as long as you can, but also realise the death is not just a waste of life, then you can say there is merit in practising meditation.

Lesson Eight

Yoga and Food

There is no right and wrong in what you eat

There is a whole plethora of foods in the human diet. If you pick a hundred people, most probably all of them will have different preferences in food.

What people eat can change dramatically according to the country, district or area they live in and therefore makes it less than straightforward in deciding on the best diet to have.

This is something that struck me when I was travelling in Africa some time ago. During my time there I visited a shop and was shocked to find it crammed full with what looked like smoked black babies hanging down from the ceiling. Later I learnt that these were in fact smoked baby monkeys which were to be torn into strips to make soup. As I went closer to smell the aroma, a pungent animal odour invaded my nostrils as if I had suddenly been put next to a cage of foxes or badgers. I realised then that something that is shocking for one person to contemplate eating is in fact perfectly natural for someone else.

There are also those who say that eating the same food everyday is better for one's health. Since animals such as elephants, cows and horses only eat grass yet are strong and fast, it is strange, they say, that human beings view eating the same food all the time as bad for the body.

If one eats the same food all the time because they feel this is what the body needs, then I cannot argue with their rationale.

Furthermore, there are those who believe that since cow's milk is designed for calves and not human beings to drink, dairy products can be harmful. Thinking about it like this, I cannot say I disagree with the logic.

Once, a person had almost persuaded me that eating sweet things was bad for the body, but I remembered reading an article in a newspaper about an elderly French woman who was a super-centenarian (over one hundred and ten years old). It mentioned how she had always loved eating chocolate everyday. Sometimes it is hard to know what to believe.

There are also those who believe that it is better to swallow food without chewing. Many may disagree with this, but also may find it hard to explain the extraordinary claims of Mao-tse Tung, who apparently practised a type of Ki training called 'Hachidankin' and strengthened his stomach by swallowing small stones.

There are furthermore those who make the unbelievable claim that it is possible to live without eating. This may be seen as a completely ludicrous statement to make, but actually in Yoga, it is believed that energy can be transferred into the body directly from light. There are apparently people in India who have survived this way without eating food for more than fifty years. No one can say for certain, therefore, that this way of living is impossible.

To conclude, since all these beliefs are right in their own way and cannot be fully dismissed, choosing what method is correct can be a confusing business.

Healthiness, a modern day affliction

I once knew a young woman who believed the slogan of a food product which stated that 'eating this product everyday will make you healthy,' a slogan which, if turned around, is effectively saying 'if you don't eat this you won't be healthy.' When the woman became ill, therefore, she believed it was because she wasn't eating the food properly, so became strict with herself and limited her diet to this food only, even taking it with her when she went on holiday. Her health then deteriorated further, leading her to question why this was happening with her strict diet regime. Her confusion, mixed with anxiety and fear, led her to fear eating any kind of food, and eventually she become neurotic.

You may think this woman foolish, but actually this kind of thing can creep up on a person easier than you think.

Here is a another similar story.

A young man was told by a clairvoyant that because of a crime he committed ten thousand years ago, he would become ill in his fortieth year. After being given this advice, he became fearful and came to me for advice on how he could prevent this from happening. His face was deadly serious.

I told him to think about the advice given to him more carefully. Ten thousand years ago would mean the time of the Altamira cave in Spain, or the Lascaux caves in France. Could he really talk about something that happened such a long time ago with such conviction?

It takes all sorts to give that sort of advice, but also all sorts to believe it, I thought to myself. I asked him if there was a reason why it was so easy for him to believe in a logic based on something which happened such a long time ago, especially since it's not unusual to get ill once or twice in one's fortieth year. 'Hmm, you've got a point there' he said, as if he had awoken from a dream.

As I meet and listen to more and more people like this I have realised that most people are governed by an clouded veil of anxiety. All of these people share a common link; they have all become mentally bound to something in order to escape from this anxiety.

The people here were cast under the spell of healthiness, health food and clairvoyance. The only advice I would give to break this spell would be 'think and live for yourself.'

The same goes for food. Before you start a diet that you hear or read about, consider first whether it suits you or not. If you find it doesn't, then avoid it even if it comes from the highest authority. After all, surely what is preferable is to enjoy what you eat and go on to live a long and healthy life as a result.

The philosophy of food in Yoga

What is the Yoga view on food?

In Yoga the body is a temple; a place where oneness with the universe can be achieved. It is therefore necessary to keep the body clean and surrounded by pure waveforms.

In order to keep your body pure by surrounding it with pure waveforms, you must follow the following points.

The method of eating in Yoga: points to remember

1-Be mindful that food gives off waveforms

Since an animal experiences fear at the moment it is killed, meat contains fear waveforms. Eating an excess amount of meat, can, therefore, act as an obstacle to meditation.

2-The waveforms of the person making the food will have an effect on the food

The waveforms and taste of a meal made by someone who is happy to make it compared to a meal made by someone who is unhappy and is making it against their will could not be more different. This is why you should try and make sure you eat food which has been lovingly prepared by someone and not churned out by a machine.

3-Do not over-eat

Over-eating is one of the main causes of unhealthiness. In Yoga, eating a small amount of food is recommended, although perhaps surprisingly, it does not say you must fast.

For most people, an appropriate amount to eat should be until your stomach is four-fifths full.

It is also important to chew well when eating. When you chew for around thirty seconds, the Peroxidase enzyme in the saliva mixes into the chewed up food, making it easy to digest. This enzyme is also known to split up carcinogens.

What should we eat?

Deciding what food is good to eat and not good to eat is a contentious issue. The many different views there are on what should be eaten only help to increase one's confusion on the matter.

On closer inspection, it could be said that this confusion is one that arises from the fact that different people are on different levels of consciousness. Someone who has a high level of consciousness from practising Yoga for a long time can tell someone of a different level of consciousness to eat what they are eating, but it may not be understood. Ultimately, therefore, I don't think you can say for certain that a particular type of food is the best.

Many of those new to Yoga start with a level of consciousness where they love eating meat. However, as they do Yoga, the amount of meat in their diet gradually decreases and they start to desire more grain and vegetables, until finally they cease to desire meat at all.

In actual fact, before I started practising Yoga, I myself loved eating meat. After practising Yoga for a while, however, my desire to drink alcohol and eat meat vanished, one after another. It had mysteriously happened that way, without any intention on my part.

My feelings on this are as follows. If you wish to eat meat, then you should do so. The same goes for alcohol. If then a change occurs within you, simply follow that change.

Nowadays, there are many healthy diets such as traditional Japanese food, wholemeal vegetarian and Macrobiotic diets, which I would advise you start thinking about eating.

By living a meditative life, you will start to develop a real taste for healthy food and will be fully satisfied with just simple food. In doing so, you will experience a lightness in body and spirit.

Although this isn't looked into much, food can be good or bad according to the state of mind of the person eating it, no matter how good the ingredients or how well prepared it is.

The most ideal way is to practise meditation before a meal. Those who do not have the time can instead say a prayer at meal time. 'I offer this food to the eternal mother of the universe,' for example, would be appropriate. Those who already say a prayer can continue with the same one.

In this way, food in Yoga is not just for preserving a state of health, but also for creating an abundance of pure waveforms. These maintain a state of purity in the temple-body which in turn leads to spiritual development.

Lesson Nine

Regain your strength with Yoga

Looking at the healing mechanism from the viewpoint of the Abo theorem

When the mind and spirit is toned through Yoga, the balance of the autonomic nerves improve and the flow of Ki (life energy) becomes stronger.

As this happens, the self-healing powers which are inherent in human beings increase. Yoga can control illnesses, even chronic ones, and can also help those who are not ill by preventing illnesses and creating an amazing level of healthiness.

The human body comprises of a vegetative part and an animal part, which are made up of vegetative nerves and animal nerves.

The vegetative nerves are in the vegetative organs such as the intestines, veins, and kidneys and make up the 'inner organ' group. The animal nerves are in the animal organs such as the muscles, nerves and outer skin and make up the 'outer layer' group.

The vegetative nerves are also called the 'autonomic' nerves. These nerves, which are not connected to the conscious mind, control many of the 'inner organ group' organs including the veins, heart, stomach, womb, bladder, endocrine gland, sweat glands, saliva glands, and pancreas.

They also automatically regulate the vegetative functions of the body. In fact, it has been discovered in recent years that the autonomic nerves control the immune system and are therefore directly linked to self-healing.

This ground breaking discovery was announced by Professor Tōru Abo of Niigata University with the Global Immunology community as a set of findings under the heading 'The control of white blood cells by the autonomic nerves.'

From the knowledge that the autonomic nerves are thus deeply connected to health and ill-health, it should be easy to understand why illnesses are cured when the body and mind is put into harmony through Yoga.

This is because Yoga is a method which strengthens and creates balance in the autonomic nerves by using the body to alternately stimulate the sympathetic nerves and para-sympathetic nerves.

The method of Yoga is special in that not only does it bring back balance in the mind and spirit and create a healthy body by improving the flow of Ki (Prana), but it also raises the spiritual level of a person.

The Autonomic nerves:

- The Sympathetic nerves

  (Breathing gets faster, heart beats faster, veins contract, blood pressure rises and stomach movement is suppressed)

- The Para-Sympathetic nerves

  (Breathing slows down, heart beat drops, veins expand, blood pressure drops, and stomach movement becomes active)

A release from illness

Modern medicine has the tendency to look for the causes of any illness, no matter how common it is, inside the body, i.e. in the abnormalities of hereditary genes. However, only three percent of illnesses are said to be due to hereditary gene abnormalities. The remainder are all due to the imbalance of the autonomic nerves.

Illnesses do not occur inside the body by accident. They happen either because of external factors or because of personal actions. Abo's theory on the the immune system states that an illness occurs because these factors disrupt the balance of the autonomic nerves.

In my opinion, Yoga is a method which finds out why the balance of the autonomic nerves have been lost and acts to restore it. Putting the mind and body in order through Yoga should, in other words, be a release from illness.

Over-use of the sympathetic nerves may cause ailments such as high blood pressure, stiff shoulders, back ache, piles, gum disease, tooth decay, dizziness, tinnitus, insomnia, uneven heartbeat, cramp, ovarian cysts, mastopathy (disease or pain of the mammary glands), and breast cancer. These ailments and illnesses occur because of prolonged over-exertion which has made the sympathetic nerves dominant.

Abo's immune system theory states that these illnesses will be cured if the para-sympathetic nerves are given more priority by removing the factor causing the over-exertion and bringing about a change in lifestyle.

Headaches are caused when either the sympathetic nerves or the para-sympathetic nerves are dominant. If you tense from stress, the sympathetic nerves become dominant, contracting the veins from the neck to the shoulders, and giving you the sort of headache where it feels your head is being squeezed. Alternatively, if there is a release of stress, the para-sympathetic nerves become dominant and can cause a surge of blood in the veins and a throbbing headache. Abo's immune system theory states that gentle exercise in relaxing the neck and shoulder muscles can be effective in curing this pain.

Furthermore, over-dominance of the para-sympathetic nerves through over-relaxing can cause allergies and swellings. People who over-use the para-sympathetic nerves can get tired quickly, dislike exercise, and feel the need to lie down after a meal. The Abo immune system theory states that the only way to remedy this is to eat moderately and reduce the over-dominance of the para-sympathetic nerves.

Yoga is recognised to be the most suitable method to cure the imbalance in the sympathetic and para-sympathetic nerves, and so remedy the ailments and illnesses I have listed above. Here are some people I know who have overcome difficult illnesses through Yoga.

Examples of people who managed to regain their health through Yoga

Mrs. A was told if she didn't have an operation immediately she would become paralysed from the waist down

A Japanese woman in London, who I will call Mrs. A, joined a tennis club after her children had all grown up, and practised tennis there every day. One day during a game, while going for the ball, she felt as if something had hit her hard in the back, and collapsed on the ground. She lay on the ground in extreme pain, unable to move or even breathe. The ambulance came and took her to hospital where it was discovered she had a herniated disc in her back.

The doctor explained that the disc cartilage had been crushed and part of it was pressing onto the nerves. It was therefore, in his opinion, necessary for surgery as soon as possible.

The woman knew friends who had undergone operations to cure back pain, yet it had either not made any difference or had in fact made the problem worse. She was therefore reluctant to follow the doctor's advice.

As she held it off, the English doctor warned her that if she didn't have the operation soon she could become paralysed from the waist down. Still unsure on what to do, the woman showed her brother, a surgeon in Tokyo, her X ray photos and asked his advice. He shared the same opinion as the doctor in London.

It was around this time that the woman came to my place, anxious and full of indecision.

My advise to her was to try out a few Yoga poses. If these didn't work, I said, she could always do the operation afterwards as a last resort.

After administering Ki therapy and reducing the pain, I introduced her to Yoga. Even though she was not able to do all the poses completely, she practised the poses with the four points (p.2-3) in mind.

Although at the start she was extremely tentative while doing the poses, she gradually became more confident. After doing this for around ten months, people around her commented with surprise on how much her health had improved. After another two months, she had recovered well enough to play tennis with her children again. More than ten years have now passed since this incident, and the woman is still enjoying good health without any problems.

The likely explanation for the woman's recovery is that the para-sympathetic nerves became dominant after relaxation in Yoga, increasing the circulation of blood to her lower back, which enabled the broken structure to repair itself. It is also likely that practising the Yoga breathing exercises improved the flow of Ki in her body, optimizing her self-healing capabilities.

In modern medicine, it seems the only way to treat a crushed disc is to remove it in an operation. In my opinion, however, merely cutting and removing a part of the human body is not the answer to the problem. It is perfectly normal for someone's bones when they get old to change shape and break. There are many elderly people out there who have good balance and are getting along fine even though their backs have become a little bent.

How Mrs. B benefited from practising Prana exercises the day after having a stroke

This story is about Mrs. B, a woman in her seventies who collapsed after having a stroke while on holiday and was taken to hospital. The day after being admitted to hospital, she started practising leg and arm Yoga poses on her bed. At the start, her legs and arms didn't do what she told them to do. In fact they felt like they belonged to someone else.

In spite of this, she persevered with the exercises everyday and slowly felt the sensation returning to her limbs. And as the sensation came back, the movement started to come back also.

When the woman was discharged from hospital, she rejoined my Yoga class. After a while she became able to do the standing on one leg pose, and is now well and living without any after effects of the stroke. Sad to say, the other three people who were with her on the ward are still undergoing rehabilitation.

I believe the fact that Mrs. B started arm and leg poses immediately after suffering her stroke (even though not told to by the doctor and nurses) was key to her miraculous recovery.

There is also no doubt that doing the arm and leg poses with a positive frame of mind improved her flow of Ki and increased blood flow in her brain which then brought out her self-healing powers and repaired the damage in her brain.

How Mrs. C overcame collagen disease with Yoga and Ki therapy

This story is about a middle-aged Japanese housewife living in London who had collagen disease and suffered a great deal of pain everyday as a result.

Although her whole body was in a great deal of pain, the left side of her neck, her shoulder, her lower back, both legs and fingertips were especially bad. Since she couldn't lie down to sleep at night because of the pain, she had to make do by sitting and leaning on cushions.

In the hope her suffering may be alleviated, the woman came to my place for Ki therapy. She was evidently very intelligent, and showed she had a comprehensive knowledge of collagen disease. Apparently, collagen disease, unlike cancer, is a disease which is relatively minor, yet difficult to treat.

The only research it has been subject to has been limited to occasional reports in medical journals, all of which she had read very carefully.

'The causes of the disease are unknown, and even though it is not immediately life-threatening like cancer, slowly the joints get more and more painful, the drugs less and less effective and the body weaker and weaker until finally anti-cancer drugs are administered and the patient dies,' she said, matter of factly.

'There is the power in the human body to cure even difficult illnesses such as this,' I replied, but the woman did not seem particularly convinced.

Every time the woman came to my place for treatment, I encouraged her not to give up, reiterating the point that there is a hidden power in the human body that is yet to be recognised by modern medicine and telling her examples of many different chronic illnesses that I had been able to treat.

At the time, the woman's hands were a deep crimson colour, as if they had been burnt. She explained that the skin had become inflamed, and that to combat this she was taking anti-inflammatory drugs.

After a number of sessions, the drugs receded, and her hands reverted back to their normal colour. As she noticed this change in her body she began to take heed of my advice. This was the turning point. Suddenly a bright light of change was lit inside her and subsequently the symptoms of her illness started to disappear as if an old skin had been shed.

The woman wanted to know how to cure her illness by herself, so I recommended to her Yoga poses that she could do by herself at home. When the woman heard 'Yoga' she was taken aback, and had good reason to be, since it is not common for Yoga to be recommended for a collagen disease sufferer who has constant pain all over the body. After I explained to her that a perfect pose is not important as long as the four points are adhered to and that the stiffer you are, the bigger the effect, she put aside her reservations and decided she would have a go.

When I had administered Ki on the woman, I showed her some simple Yoga poses and breathing exercises which we practised together. After we had done this she mentioned how she had enjoyed the relaxing pose at the end. From then on, this Yoga and Ki lesson became a regular occurrence.

After a year or so, the woman told me that she would like to attend my Yoga class. I was delighted with her positive attitude. She had improved her health so much that no one at the Yoga class suspected her of having collagen disease. At present she is a devoted student and more full of life than the average person.

Lesson Ten

Yoga treatment can work against chronic illnesses such as cancer

Healing Power from Within

Curing an illness is possible either through treatment or healing. Treatment is administered from outside the body, while healing occurs from within.

Modern medicine's standard treatment of cancer is from the outside and involves cutting out as many cancerous cells as possible, using anti-cancer drugs and radiation to eliminate any which remain. It is, in other words, a triple-pronged treatment of surgical operation, anti-cancer drugs and radiation.

In my view there is a limit to how far this triple-pronged treatment can go. Administering anti-cancer drugs and radiation to a patient who is already weak from an operation is like kicking a man when he is down. It lowers the energy in the body and weakens the immune system further.

At this stage, the only option left is to use the healing power from within. Using this healing power to cure an illness is the main focus of what is called Alternative therapy. The term Alternative therapy is used to describe all the alternative methods to modern medicine. These include Ayuvedic medicine, Chiropracty, Acupuncture, Kampo (Chinese herbal remedies), Image creation therapy, Dietary treatment, Massage and Ki therapy.

Professor Abo says that cancer is an illness which has an extreme restricting effect on the immune system but that this effect can always be cured by reducing the stress caused by tension of the sympathetic nerves and re-invigorating the para-sympathetic nerves.

The Abo theory on the immune system states that continued tension of the sympathetic nerves are not only detrimental to blood circulation and bowel movement, but also lead to an increase in the number of granulocyte white blood cells which release active oxygen and protect against outside enemies such as bacteria. When this active oxygen from the granulocytes accumulates in the body, it becomes the basis of tissue damage. As the tissue is damaged and repaired, the surrounding cells start to change the DNA, creating cancer cells.

It is therefore, according to Professor Abo, the increase in granulocytes which lead to the creation of cancer cells.

In order to reduce the number of granulocyte white blood cells it is necessary to suppress the sympathetic nerves and reinvigorate the para-sympathetic nerves, which will increase the number of lympa cells and strengthen the immune system. In his book 'Changing your diet to improve your immune system and avoid illness' (Nagaoka shoten), Professor Abo states the importance of escaping from the fear of cancer, listing four methods. He says that if you think cancer is scary and incurable then your immune system will weaken, but if you hold a prepared and relaxed mind, your immune system will strengthen and stop the spread of the disease.

How to heal cancer yourself

Up till now, I have treated many people with cancer and have witnessed some dramatically overcome the disease. In my view, therefore, it is not an incurable disease. When I see patients left hairless from chemotherapy and very weak from radiation and evasive surgery, I wonder, especially after reading Professor Abo's research, whether cancer is so terrible as to warrant such drastic measures. I wonder why this treatment has to be undertaken by all cancer sufferers in spite of the suffering involved, considering that even after all the suffering, more people die than survive. The belief that cancer is a truly terrifying disease and so worthy of even the most extreme of treatments is something that has, I believe, become a universal and incontestable fact in the minds of doctors.

I believe cancer can be cured, by changing the way you think and live, and by having the strong belief that you can cure your own illness by yourself. There is a book that made an impression on me called 'A cancer treatment which gives hope' (Michio Saitō, Shūeisha shinsho) in which a television producer reports on various people who have miraculously overcome cancer without resorting to modern medicine's three-pronged treatment of surgery, chemotherapy and radiation therapy.

I will list now some points to remember for healing cancer by yourself. Some are from my experiences of treating cancer and some are from the book.

1-If you get cancer, believe that it can be cured

Thinking in this way gives birth to hope. Cancer can be cured even when it is not diagnosed and treated early. This natural healing is called 'natural regression.' As the immune system gets stronger, it can have the effect of making five millimetres to one centimetre of cancerous cells disappear. It has apparently also been possible for cancer to disappear in this way even when it has grown to four or five centimetres.

2-Accept that you are responsible for contracting cancer

Cancer is something that is created by yourself. It is not something that has latched onto your body from the outside. It is therefore necessary to accept responsibility for the cancer so that you can cure it by yourself.

3-Change your lifestyle

Negative factors such as overwork, irregular lifestyle, smoking, obesity and lack of exercise can all contribute to developing cancer. Treating your body well, therefore, may help revert the process and make the cancer disappear.

4-Improve your Diet

It is important to moderate your intake of meat, not to overeat, to moderate salt, fat and sugar intake, and to eat a healthy and balanced diet by, for example, eating wholemeal rice and vegetables.

5-Keep your mind in shape

Do not to keep stress building up inside. Instead of being anxious about things, it is necessary to have a direct and positive outlook on life. It is also important to feel gratitude. If you practise Yoga properly, and not just as an exercise, your anxieties will naturally die down. Those who suffer from a lot of stress have a low immune system. By relaxing in Yoga, their immune system will become stronger.

6-Be confident that you can cure your illness on your own

It is important to realise that by changing your lifestyle, you can cure your illness by yourself, and that the role of the doctor is only to assist you. You can overcome cancer by achieving what is possible to do on your own.

7-Choose to do nothing

Even if you leave the cancer as it is, you will not immediately die. This is why, as Professor Abo advocates, you must have the courage to take only the minimal amount of drugs and surgery so your body does not lose too much strength.

If you have been told that you have terminal cancer, then it would be hard to hold up the schedule of the three pronged treatment once the wheels are in motion. If possible, however, try and get a second and third opinion, and think long and hard about the treatment before going ahead with it.

It is a valid option to leave the cancer as it is. There are those who have lived with terminal cancer for ten to fifteen years and even those who have had a natural remission without having surgery or drugs. Some people come to the realisation that this very moment is the apex of their lives, and cease to have regrets about the past since they have lived their life how they wanted to up till now. With that realisation they either continue living with their cancer, or see their cancer go into remission.

8-When choosing a type of alternative therapy, pick one which suits you best

Since cancer is uniquely personal like the face, it follows that alternative therapy must be also. Just because a treatment works for Mr. A does not mean it will work for Mr. B or Mr. C. In actual fact, that is what makes cancer so difficult to treat. The thing is to find a method that suits you best. How much you pay for it does not equate to how effective it will be.

9-Choose an alternative therapy which feels the best

If it doesn't feel good, you won't be able to relax. If you can't relax, your immune system will not improve.

10-Be cheerful

One thing in particular which all of these people who overcame cancer have in common is their positive attitude. Choose to be cheerful and sustain this feeling. If you get depressed, think of a way in which you can rise up and become cheerful again.

I will now introduce some effective self-healing methods.

Image healing with the mantra 'I will be cured'

Here is a story of a man from the book 'A cancer treatment which gives hope.' He was in a desperate situation; his malignant cell indicator continued to rise even after half his large intestine, and half of his kidney in a follow up operation, was removed. In this situation he tried the following image healing method.

He imagined himself getting better and repeated the words 'I will be cured' aloud to himself everyday.

Every morning he would sing 'I will be cured, I will be cured' while going for a walk, and repeated these words throughout the day.

In this way, he started to believe that he would be cured, not in his head, but in his body.

As he repeated this everyday so that his body started to believe it too, the cancer started to change. Five years after his first operation, his malignant cell indicator has regressed into a stable and safe level and his cancer has not increased or spread.

The Coué method

This is a method started by the French psychotherapist Emille Coué (1857-1926). All it involves is repeating the phrase, 'day by day, in every way, I am getting better and better' over and over again to yourself. Apparently many people with incurable diseases have been cured with this amazingly simple method.

The Simonton method

This is a healing program for cancer as devised by the American professor Carl Simonton. It is a form of image healing, so those who are good at using their imagination please have a go.

Sit with your eyes closed. Now imagine the healthy cells eating all the bad cells in the body and repeat this over and over again.

Picture this behind the eyelids as if looking at a screen. Make it as vivid as possible.

Illness curing breathing exercise (Sōnen[1] breathing exercise)

This breathing exercise was introduced in the 'Japan psychic science society' journal by Doctor Nobuo Shioya, under the title 'Steady mind, steady breathing' exercise. I have practised it myself.

I recommend it to all sorts of people suffering from various illnesses and it has proved very effective. I have therefore chosen to rename it 'the illness curing' breathing exercise (Sōnen breathing exercise).

1- Sit in the 'Seiza' pose. For those who find this difficult, sit cross-legged, or on a chair, making sure your back is straight. Bend your elbows at right angles and keep them at the side of your body. Interlock the fingers and shape the palms of your hands as if holding a ball.

2- Breathe in from the crown of your head (Hyakue tsubo) to the tanden (area below the stomach). Believe that the infinite energy of the universe has come into your tanden.

3- Hold your breath when you have finished the inhalation. Tense your stomach and constrict your sphincter muscles, putting pressure on the tanden.

For those who have an illness: While holding your breath, declare 'My (name of illness) is now cured.' Do not say 'please may it be cured'; the declaration is important.

4- Exhale slowly from the nose. Say to yourself, 'All the old and stagnant energy has left the body,' and end the exhalation.

---

[1]   'Sōnen' is focus on a positive mental image.

Breathe in now through the nose.

5- Take a normal breath, and if you have an illness, imagine yourself healthy again.

Practice the cycle from 2-5 twenty-five times in a day. You can divide it into ten in the morning and fifteen in the evening if you wish.

For those with numerous illnesses, practise it twenty-five times for each illness.

6- When you have finished, breathe normally ten times and relax. Imagine yourself healthy again.

Illness curing meditation technique (Nanso method)

This is the meditation method used by the monk Hakuin, called the 'Nanso' method.

In the reign of the fifth Tokugawa Shogun Tsunayoshi, the great Hakuin was a monk of the Rinzai sect of Zen Buddhism. He had developed a 'Zen disease' as a result of undertaking extreme training when he was young. Today, this illness may be described as a type of neurosis. It is said that he obtained this knowledge from a 'sennin'[2] living in the mountains and that it cured him of his illness. The 'nan' of 'nanso' means 'soft' and the 'so' is boiled milk which has hardened into butter or cheese.

1- Sit in the Lotus or Half-lotus pose. It is also fine to sit on a chair. Rest both hands on your knees.

2- Imagine that a soft egg-size ball of cream is sitting on the crown of your head.

3- Imagine that the temperature of your head melts this cream, giving off a pleasant aroma.

---

[2]   A 'sennin' is a mystical hermit who lives in the mountains.

4- Imagine that this melted cream seeps into your head and cleanses all the impurities as it descends from your neck into the tips of your fingers.

5- Now imagine this fragrant cream seeping down from your neck to your chest, and each individual organ in the stomach region. Imagine the cream washing away all the impurities as it does so. Imagine the cream descending right down to the coccyx bone.

6- From the coccyx bone, imagine the cream descending into and washing all the impurities in your thighs, knees and calves, before finally coming out of the soles of the feet.

Repeat 2 to 6.

Afterword

After the release of my book 'The Power of Life' (Heibonsha, Author House), many people contacted me to find out more about Yoga.

While 'The Power of Life' was more observational, this book is specifically about how to practise Yoga and Ki.

As I mentioned in the chapter 'Yoga and food,' in Japan at the moment the sheer number of differing reports on what is good and what is bad for you make it very difficult to know exactly what to believe. As I'm writing this sentence now, I can see on today's newspaper a headline, 'What is the best type of water to drink?'

The article, by Professor Takeo Samaki of the Science education department in Doshisha Women's College, states that water claiming to cure specific illnesses with the labels 'water clusters (molecular groups), waveforms, minus ions' should not be trusted.

There is also the article by Professor Emeritus Koichiro Fujita of the Parasitology department of the Tokyo medical and dental college who responds to the question 'what is the most delicious water?' by saying, 'taste is a very subjective thing. I would say that whatever water you are used to drinking and which is cold is probably the best.' (Both articles are from the 20th December 2006 edition of the Asahi Newspaper).

Furthermore, in the health section of the Asahi.com website, I read an article with the headline, 'Ministry of Health, Labour and Welfare research on 60,000 people shows that constipation and cancer of the large intestine is unrelated' (20th Dec 2006).

The article read, 'As reported in an American medical journal, the popular belief that cancer of the large intestine and constipation are related due to the harmful agents in faecal matter staying in the intestines for a long period of time is refuted by the immunology research carried out by the Ministry of Health, Labour and Welfare research institute (led by the head of the National cancer prevention centre research department, Shoichiro Tsugane).'

As new information such as this continues to enter our daily lives it only serves to confuse us. Should we, for example, buy mini cluster, minus ion or waveform water or worry about getting intestinal cancer from constipation?

In the midst of this chaotic daily influx of information I remember a quotation of Buddha.

'You are the only master. Who else? Subdue yourself and discover your master.' (The Dhammapada)

Before you start getting pulled around by all the different kinds of information, I think it is important remember the following three points.

- Before accepting what someone tells you, think about it carefully first.

- Accept something which feels right for you, otherwise disregard it.

- You are you and others are others. Others can never become you. Think, therefore, about creating a way of living without copying how other people live theirs.

I believe what is required for us to do right now is, as Buddha says, to control the self, the master of who you are. We can achieve this now by training the body and mind through methods such as Yoga and Ki therapy, methods I hope, will serve as more than just a present-day fad.

To end, I would like to express my deepest thanks to Fumiyo Watanabe and Atsuko Otsu for their help, Shō Shirota for the book design, Fusako Komine for the illustration, Takashi Takaoka from Heibonsha and everyone else who contributed to the publication of this book.

2007—At home in London.
Isamu Mochizuki

Reference

Yoga konpon kyoten (transl: The basic Yoga Sutras) (Tsuruji Sahoda, Hirakawa Publishers)

Kaisetsu Yoga Sutra (transl: Understanding Yoga Sutras) (Tsuruji Sahoda, Hirakawa Publishers)

Yoga, Yoga Gyōhō no dankaiteki shūrenhō ((transl: Yoga, Step by step Yoga training) (Kazuo Banba, Hirakawa Publishers)

Inochi no chikara (Isamu Mochizuki, Heibonsha Publishers), (The Power of Life (english translation), Isamu Mochizuki, Author House publishers)

Kōsureba byōki wa naoru (transl: Do this and your illness will disappear) (Tōru Abo, Shinchō sensho)

Kibō no ganchiryō (transl: A cancer treatment which gives hope) (Michio Saitō, Shūeisha shinsho)

Ki, Meiso, Yoga no kenkōgaku (transl: The health sciences of Ki, Meditation and Yoga) (Hiroshi Motoyama, Meichokankokai)

Kikō, chūgoku hiden no kenkōhō (transl: Kikō, China's secret health method) (Baseball magazine company, Chūgoku, Jinmin Taiiku Publishers)

Zusetsu Kikōhō (transl: Illustrated guide to Kikō therapy) (Minoru Hoshino and Takashi Tsumura, Hakujyusha)

Yuishiki no susume (transl: Writings on the Vijnapti Matrata) (Moriya Okano, NHK Publishing)

Aru Yogi no Jijoden (Autobiography of a Yogi) (Paramahansa Yogananda, Morikita Publishers)

Zusetsu Bukkyogo Daijiten (transl: Illustrated Dictionary of Buddhist terminology) (Hajime Nakamura, Tokyo Shoseki)

Krishnamurti no meisōroku (transl: Krishnamurti on meditation) (translated by Junichi Ōno, Sunmark Bunko)

Tōru Abo Byōki ni naranai menekiryoku wo tsukuru mainichi no shokuji (transl: Tōru Abo- How to build a strong immune system and avoid illness with food) (Tōru Abo, supervised by Keiko Sugimoto, Nagaoka Shoten)

Buddha no hito to shisō (transl: Buddhist people and thinking) (Hajime Nakamura, Shōji Tanabe, NHK books)

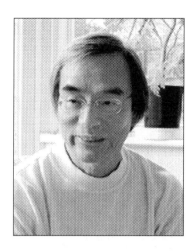

About the Author

Isamu Mochizuki

Born in 1948, in Shizuoka Prefecture. In 1973, at the age of 25, he moved to London. From there, he travelled many countries in Europe, joined a Kibbutz in Israel, and travelled the Sinai Peninsula. He then travelled by land through Greece, the Middle East, Turkey, Afghanistan, Nepal and India where he contracted acute hepatitis and had to return back to Japan.

In 1979 he again went to London. The following year he travelled by land to Africa where he lived rough and hitch-hiked for seven months through various countries. During his time there he also climbed Mount Kilimanjaro and traversed the Sahara desert. While doing so he started to understand intuition and let it guide him in his daily life.

In 1980, he started learning Shorinji Kempo, Ki therapy and Yoga by himself, which opened the world of Ki up to him. In 1986, while in Africa, he discovered that he had the power to heal other people. In 1987, he went to India to undertake training, and was initiated into the secrets of Yoga in the Himalayan mountains from a guru. He visited Sai Baba's ashram and many Yoga practises all over India.

In 1988, he deepened his understanding of Ki with the late founder of 'Wadō,' Sōho Hayakawa in Kanazawa. After this he set up a Yoga class and Ki-therapy clinic in London which he continues to this present day.

As an author, he has written in Japanese a travelogue of his time in the Sinai Peninsula called 'Seinen to Sabaku' (transl: 'The Youth and the Desert,' Kodansha Service centre, 2002), a collection of poems entitled, 'Hokumei' (transl: 'Northern Providence') (Kadokawa Shoten, 2003), Inochi no Chikara ('The Power of Life,' Heibonsha, 2004), and a conversation with the writer Hiroyuki Itsuki entitled 'Ki no Hakken' (transl: 'Discovering Ki,' Heibonsha, 2004).

His book 'Inochi no Chikara' was translated into English and is published by Author House with the title 'The Power of Life.'

About the Translator

Simon Grisdale

Based in London. Graduated from London University Japanese department in 2006. During University, he damaged his spinal cord in an accident and became confined to a wheelchair. He discovered Yoga and Ki therapy at that time and after some years of recuperation, became involved in translation. He also started playing the piano again since his music scholarship at school. In 2011 he won the Concours de Grand Amateurs piano competition in Paris and now plays various recitals. As well as this book, he has translated 'The Power of Life' by Isamu Mochizuki.